I0413072

Mindful Eating:

Free Yourself from the Diet Language

Ayelet Kalter

Copyright © 2015
by Ayelet Kalter
All rights reserved
ISBN: 1511611219
ISBN-13: 978-1511611213

TO MY CLIENTS

ACKNOWLEDGMENTS

There are moments in life, that you look at yourself and you are overwhelmed with bliss. Such emotion you cannot state in words, but is clearly some kind of grace. This is how I feel when I turn to thank those who walk beside me for many years. Each in its own special way, being who he is to me. Not because they have written a word in the book, have read it or would read. But because the way they listen to me, think with me, and sometimes feel me.

There is no special order to their place in this list, but they play a special role in my life: Professor Zamir Halpern, Eli Gonen, Dr. Zeev Weiner and Hanoch Dovrat.

A special place is reserved for a dear woman, Avishag Lewkowicz, who, with modesty and faith, accompany me for many years in my not so simple way. I love her presence beside me. And to make this list complete, I'll add my little loving familly's members.

For all of those – thank you.

Ayelet

ACKNOWLEDGMENTS

CONTENTS

INTRODUCTION- WHAT IS THE PROBLEM?

For many years I have helped people in their attempts to lose weight. I firmly believed that this was possible. Since 1984, for almost 15 years, I managed, as a certified clinical dietitian, one of the busiest clinics in Israel. The achievements I witnessed were impressive; patients were satisfied. But at the same time, I began noticing a troubling pattern. Over the years, many patients continued tracking fluctuations in their weight, and I noticed a strange pattern: most of the patients did lose weight, but nearly all of them regained it. This raised a lot of questions for me, which drove me to expand my professional knowledge.

My first significant step was attending a conference about treating eating disorders held in Philadelphia. I vividly recall one experience I had there. We had gathered for a two day workshop with twenty five professionals, most of them psychologists specializing in treating eating disorders. The workshop was hosted by a group of women, members of the American "Fat Acceptance" movements. They were particularly heavy women. During the workshop, we were asked to get up and dance in a circle. Twenty five women ranging all weights and sizes danced. Only me, who was the thinnest, didn't dare stand up. I was so ashamed of my body, I felt utterly embarrassed.

It was a rattling experience. I suddenly realized that slimness does not insure self-confidence. The heavy women danced with a light step, their self-confidence a stark contrast to my insecurity, opened a door for me. I stepped through it and embarked on a personal and professional journey, one which passed through dozens of conventions and workshops abroad. At some of these I was a featured speaker, at others I was a regular participant. These conventions and workshops included formal studies in a variety of disciplines: family and couples therapy, Buddhism with a therapeutic point of view, group leading, and psychodynamic approaches to understanding adult development to name but a few.

After conducting extensive research, I realized there are no subjects or fields of research that aren't in some way linked with the existential issue of food and eating. Sociology and politics, motifs in literature and poetry, in cinema, in Judaism, and in different social situations. This issue is also directly linked to social conceptions about thinness, as well as the beauty myth, cognitive psychology, psychodrama and Buddhism. All of these are contexts within which we can understand our eating patterns. Government policy, the right to invade the individual's domain, weight and health discrimination are contributing factors as well. All of these have made the issue of obesity weightier than a proper body mass index or the number of pounds being read out on a scale.

My research compelled me to leave the dietetic profession in favor of a new, complex, and amazingly effective approach: Helping people with their relationship with food they eat.

This book is not another diet book which pretends to reveal the gospel of staying thin. It is also not a book devoted to social and political criticism of the diet industry. Dieting and battling weight gain is a substantial issue in the lives of millions. It is also a major source of inner conflict. My objective is not to argue with reality, but to use it as a base of knowledge for the argument that forms the backbone of this book: how battling against weight gain and striving for slimness hurts people by disrupting eating habits and causes an ongoing conflict between people and their bodies.

In the last fifty years, as a result of the war on fat and mostly because of its failure, a new language about diet has developed. I shall refer to this as the Diet Language. This language can be found around the globe, and is one that judges a person's value, social status and health in terms of his or her body weight. In this culture, people count their calories and struggle with guilt and fear about their food consumption.

In this book I present a different eating language, "Mindful Eating". This approach will snap the chains of the old diet culture which bind you to its rules and language. My call to you is not "Let us be fat," however, but "Let's accept what we cannot change about our bodies in order to change what we can." What Mindful Eating offers us is simply a return to sane eating which normalizes the way we eat and how we feel about our bodies regardless of our body weight. Within the human race, there exists a natural and legitimate diversity in body shape and weight. Recognizing this diversity and acknowledging the eating patterns specific to each one of us could help make our lives freer, and surprisingly more healthy and valuable too.

In Webster's dictionary, obesity is defined as "an excessive accumulation of fat." But an excess of fatty tissue is what increases the risk of disease, not necessarily excess weight. Contrary to popular belief, obesity is not a disease which is measured in pounds but in the function of fat cells. Even so, the most common method in the world to measure obesity is by the Body Mass Index (BMI) which is calculated as body weight (in pounds) divided by height (in inches) squared. Today the BMI levels are determined by the following scale:

- Dangerously thin (underweight)- less than 18.5
- Normal body weight- 18.5 to 24.9
- Overweight- 25 to 29.9
- Obesity, grade 1 obesity- 30 to 34.9
- Grade 2 and 3 obesity, morbidly obese- 35 and over

The main advantage of the BMI scale is that it's easy to calculate. Its main drawback is that it doesn't take into account age, gender, ethnicity, body type and fat distribution, and does not distinguish between muscle tissue and fat tissue. In fact, it is not a reliable measurer of fat mass and the way it is dispersed in the body.

Since the late twentieth century, it is becoming clearer in professional circles that weight gain cannot be linked automatically with illness, and there are more reliable and efficient measures than the BMI scale to predict physical health. Fat percentages, waist circumference, and the ratio between waist and hip circumference are now considered in professional circles as better predictors of health and life expectancy than the Body Mass Index scale, but they are not enough. And still the hegemony of the Body Mass Index- and the entire culture bound within this measure-continues to reign over the public.

According to data from the World Health Organization (WHO), obesity, as defined by the BMI measure, is a global epidemic from which over a billion people are suffering. Apocalyptic forecasts predict that by the year 2030, most of the world's population will suffer from it.

In the U.S, about 64% of the adult population is defined as overweight or obese, meaning over 30 in the BMI scale . And in Israel, according to data issued by the Israel Center for Disease Control –ICDC and Israel National Health Interview Survey – INHIS-2 from 2007-2010 shows that about 41% of men and 30% of women are overweight by BMI standards (weighted by population group and age) and about 15.2% of men and 15.7% of women are obese. A report published by the Ministry of Health in November 2013 states over half of the Israeli population is overweight or obese.

Obesity, and especially abdominal obesity, is part of the metabolic syndrome which manifests itself in low levels of HDL cholesterol, a high concentration of triglycerides, elevated blood pressure and disorder in blood sugar levels while fasting. As such, it puts one at risk of many chronic diseases, including heart disease, fatty liver, sleep apnea, and different kinds of cancer. It is also associated with the progression of type 2 diabetes (which is also one of the constantly rising epidemics of the 21st Century).

The connection between obesity and diabetes has created the term "Diabesity," which links these two epidemics together. Today obesity is considered a chronic disease[1] and it is categorized as such in the International Classification of Diseases (ICD-9). According to this approach, we find that obesity is linked to disease more than smoking, alcoholism, and poverty is. Following these findings, a comprehensive public campaign is in play led by health groups all over the world against the global obesity epidemic, even though many findings paint a much more complicated picture which raises questions about the general assumption that being obese is an illness or helps cause it.

This all-encompassing intimidation campaign encourages a war against obesity that has become in many senses a war against people who are affected by obesity. Many studies show negative attitudes directed towards people because of their weight, and they clearly show that such unfair discrimination is growing. A man or a woman affected by weight issues is judge as being responsible for his or her weight. Body weight is also is perceived as having attributes like ugliness, emotional disorders, moral flaws, lack of control, negligence, lack of willpower, irrationality, noisiness, dirtiness, laziness, loneliness, and giving in to cravings. Such characteristics provoke repulsion, contempt, and condescension. In 2015, being fat means bearing a mark of disgrace. A successful diet is a testament of respect, ability, control, perseverance, and success and a slim body the testament of a strong and worthy personality. A body which is fat is perceived as "broken" and in need of being fixed. And it can be fixed. According to this perception, a person is not born fat but becomes fat. This argument further claims that inside every fat person hides a thin person, so with a precise diet and psychological process, the thin person hiding within the fat one will emerge.

This perception, as I have learned over the years, not only doesn't help those struggling with weight, but causes or intensifies suffering. It ignores natural human diversity and harbors needless cruelty. In any case, it does not fulfill its promise- in the long run, people do not become thinner than they are.

This book will suggest to you a different approach and a different language of eating, offering an alternative approach to the Diet Language and the weight centered approaches behind it. This is a health centered approach and not a weight centered one, and the eating language accompanying it will be called: Mindful Eating. This approach is based on current studies which disconnect the simplistic connections made between weight and illness and between personal value and body weight. It bases itself on a vast world of thought- the essence of which is the meeting point between Buddhism and advanced approaches in cognitive psychology- and gives us a plethora of tools which can help improve our knowledge of ourselves as a whole, not just in relation to our body weight.

The language of Mindful Eating includes some liberating (and revolutionary) notions, but it is not easy to accept. I invite you to take a deep breath and open your heart and mind to it.

Weight gain has not always been abominable. We have not always been slaves to the pursuit of thinness. In the Middle Ages, thinness was a symbol of low social status, poverty, and disease, while an accumulation of body fat was perceived as a sign of strength, health, and high social status. Painters illustrated this in their paintings. Rubens, Botticelli, Rembrandt, Gauguin, and Matisse often drew full figured women. They saw them as a symbol of beauty, fertility, and vivaciousness.

In the 19th century, during the Victorian Era, a piece of clothing called a corset reigned supreme. The corset was made to rein in the woman's body and create an hourglass figure. The corset was the seed from which the social belief that a thin figure was ideal grew. This belief began to take deeper root in the 1920's, when slim figures and narrow waists became the ideal beauty for women. Women perceived the thin look as symbolizing freedom and liberty. Modernization and the industrial era churned out mass produced clothes in set sizes (unlike the clothes previously tailored for every person by their own sizes), and the woman who did not fit into the set sizes painfully learned she must change. Thus the restrictions on a woman's body passed from the physical bonds of a corset to the invisible bonds of social mores.

The roots of the medical theory linking weight with ill health can be found in the late 19th and early 20th centuries. The responsibility for it lies with American insurance companies, who have spent years searching for a way to predict early mortality in order to increase their profits from life insurance. They were looking for an objective, convenient, and inexpensive measure that could signal an increased mortality risk. Body weight provided a fitting parameter. This resulted in weight and height charts which first appeared in 1897 and lasted until 1983. They later served as the basis for the ideal body weight recommendations expressed in the Body Mass Index. The term "overweight" referred to body weight above the recommended range, and the assumption was that the risk of disease and mortality increased when body weight was 20% than recommended. The insurance companies then used the weight numbers to create a payment scale for insured customers who were panicked because of their body weight and the supposed risks of illness and early mortality associated with it.

A key player in this story was Dr. Brandreth Symonds, who headed the medical department of the Mutual Life

Insurance Company in New York. In an article published in 1909 in *McClure's Magazine*, he wrote, "The excessive weight, whether it consists of fat or muscle, is not a pool of reserves giving strength to the body, but a burden which must be nourished, if muscle, and that markedly interferes with nutrition and function, if fat."

Between 1890 and 1909 about 12 articles were published about weight gain. In the following two decades over a hundred articles were published, with titles like "Get Rid of That Fat" and "Fat and Fatality." The message that began spreading over the world was "Watching your weight is a worthy goal, and it may be a question of life and death." By this stage, America was already deep into the first round of the pursuit of the elimination of "excess" body weight.

At the same time, doctors continued seeing many patients who were sick with infectious diseases triggered by being too thin.

Dr. Louis Dublin was responsible for starting the next stage of the campaign against body weight. The head biologist and statistician in the Metropolitan Life Insurance Company, Dublin established the undisputed belief that weight gain was the world's primary source of illness and premature mortality. At a large medical conference held in the U.S. in 1951, Dublin announced that men suffering from marked obesity were at a 70% higher risk of mortality than men of average weight. What drew the doctors' attention was his claim that weight gain could lead to mortality especially in light of the significant decline in deaths from tuberculosis and pneumonia- diseases common among people of low weight. Dublin went on to claim that contrary to what was commonly believed in the past, there was no longer any benefit in heavy weight as a protective measure in young age- but quite the opposite. Curiously, Dublin was the one who warned a number of years earlier that underweight individuals under thirty years of age were at risk of premature mortality. This time he declared that If in the past health risks were attributed only to morbid obesity, today even those slightly overweight are at risk. In one stroke, Dublin alleged that millions of people were at possible risk- and enlarged the insurance companies' profit potential. Researchers who later tried to reexamine his findings failed.

Dublin is known as the man who coined the term "ideal body weight." According to his perception that the human body did not experience natural weight fluctuations, Dublin believed that the body weight a person has at the age of twenty five is ideal, and every effort should be made to sustain it throughout the rest of his or her life. If so, how must we sustain our ideal body weight? By dieting, of course. And indeed, in 1951, an ad campaign against weight gain was launched in the U.S. funded by the government, the medical establishment, and the insurance companies. The establishment declared that excess weight is a decisive risk factor of heart disease, kidney disease, diabetes, and cancer, and that obesity among adults was a result of overeating. The message to Americans was "Eat Less!"

Dieting soon became the primary weapon in the war against fat, and it was only natural that nutritionists joined the battle as an inseparable part of the thin campaign. The ideal weight listed in weight and height charts became what many people desired. Over the years, it got lower and lower. Absurdly, the ideal weight that was set was considerably lower than the population's average body weight, and most people had to starve themselves in order to reach it. So, the number of overweight people joining the dieting circle gradually increased. Despite Dublin's claim that America is simply too fat," and despite the weight loss campaigns and scare tactics, America was not losing weight. And surprisingly, Americans were healthier, and morbidity decreased.

Meanwhile, the fashion industry continued to shift towards thin as the ideal body image. In 1947 Christian Dior presented a new look for women's clothing- a slim and narrow style that for most women was a mere fantasy. In the sixties, the waifish model Twiggy continued to symbolize the transition from a voluptuous womanly figure to a boyish one: in other words, a woman-child. And indeed, the joining of forces between the insurance companies and the fashion industry inspired a new message: not only is body fat unhealthy, it is also unfashionable.

Mass media signed on to the campaign, and a new axiom was born: beautiful, healthy, sexy, happy people – especially those of status and power- are thin people. Thin sold everything: cars, clothes, bags, shoes, and also…food. Paying no heed, people of all ages and races were unwittingly becoming slaves to the thin ideal.

1985 marked the beginning of the next stage in the anti-fat campaign that led to obesity as being defined as the plague of the western world. Obesity research centers and facilities to treat the problem were established all around the world. Weight loss seminars were held, periodicals devoted to fitness appeared on newsstands, and the anti-fat message was spread around the professional community and the general public. All of this was funded by financiers with an interest in escalating the medicalization of human behavior. A process where a certain behavior is defined as a medical problem or illness, and the person characterized by this behavior is defined as in need of treatment. And the campaign took off. If, early on, weight gain was considered the result of more calories consumed than burned, today it is associated with countless factors including birth weight, gender, race, genetics, obese parents, living in cities, using a car, low income, low education, single families, eating in front of the television, avoiding physical activity, eating in school, using vending machines, lack of family dinners, buying processed food, eating fast food… the list is endless.

Obesity was mentioned in the International Classification of Diseases Book(ICD-9) and was officially declared a disease in 1991. From that moment on, an entire industry has evolved which surrounds it with medicine, treatments, and surgeries that have many beneficiaries: medical professionals and academics, government and public health officials, the pharmaceutical industry, the sports industry, and the diet industry. The diet industry and the pharmaceutical industry subsidize studies headed by researchers from the world's leading research institutes, which eventually lead to the production of new products and treatments designed to help promote the belief that thinness equates health.

The world into which we are born lives, breathes, demands, and promises thinness. It promises a new and better life to those who achieve it. It barrages us with success stories which claim thinness is a wonderful thing. Everyone longs for it. The chase after thinness is akin to chasing after the golden lottery ticket. Millions buy it, but only one wins. And millions continue to buy into the fantasy of perfect thinness and the happiness that they believe will come with it. As long as we go on feeling dissatisfied with our body, someone will recognize it and want to make money from it. There is enormous interest, both open and concealed, that the fear of being fat will become so deep rooted, that there will be nearly no one who is capable of loving themselves as they are.

An example of the way in which these messages are communicated can be seen in the marketing of one of the American weight loss diet companies. The company placed "before and after" pictures on the home page of their website with the tagline "I finally got my life back- I'm myself again." This company which claims to help people lose weight does not stop at thinness; it also claimes to give life back. And not just any life, but "Your life." A quick glance shows how much weight the woman in the picture lost and our thoughts automatically create the connection between the beauty she acquired when she lost weight and the claim this woman got her life "back." These pictures etch into our minds the simplistic message "Weight loss gives back life." And this is generally not stated a question or thought, but as a fact. Such advertisements gives us certainty, not doubt, and makes us believe a new diet myth: losing weight is crucial to controlling your life. The diet industry sells and we, who must be thin- buy. A Google search under "diet products" points to nearly 5 million results. Global Weight Watchers earned 4 billion dollars in 2007 from their products and services.

Jenny Craig, another dieting mogul, reported revenue of 558 million dollars in 2007. And indeed, her website doesn't say "Jenny Craig helps you lose weight," it says "Jenny Craig- We change lives." This is your opportunity to be happy, to change your life, to buy the magic. Who can resist such fabulous claims?

In many senses, the strive for thinness has become a sort of religion, complete with its own rituals and beliefs. Like any religion, practicing it gives meaning to life and becomes the ultimate goal that acts as a beacon for many people. The ideal of thinness on one hand and fear of gaining weight on the other have become embedded into our social consciousness. This[2] has lead to:

- The myths about a wonderful future life awaiting those who succeed in becoming thin.
- Role models such as celebrities and fitness gurus (iconographies) who can be admired and mimicked. People who provide inspiration and hope of "a more promising" future.
- Rituals meant to organize daily life: calorie counting, food diaries, weigh ins, obsessive physical activity, and cooking special "diet" foods.

- Rules stating what food to avoid and how to do so, and how much to eat and when.
- Create moral rules and a judgmental language. Outlines good and bad foods. Allowed and forbidden. You're "bad" if you eat ice cream. You're "good" if you eat a salad. The rules, following or not following them, become the system with which a person judges himself and assesses his worth and punishes or rewards himself accordingly.
- Created communities of people through the way in which they eat, diet, gain weight, and lose weight by dieting.
- Promises "happiness" at the end of the road. Happiness that relies on thinness, embodying perfection.

And again, I will mention that this was not how things have always been. Up until two decades ago, body regimenting was mostly about women. Susie Orbach, a British psychologist, in her book "*Fat is a Feminist Issue*", published in the seventies, marked the harbinger of revealing an issue that has grown worse with the years: the definition of a woman through her body. Orbach's breakthrough was not only in bringing to light the physical terms, fat, thin, and overweight but in emphasizing the emotional depth at the base of the use of these terms. The term "fat", Orbach showed us, does not deal with only the physical body, but with a state of mind.

Susie Orbach illustrated well the difficulty in expressing emotions and the way we avoid feeling them through eating or abstaining from it. She pointed to the connection, which has now become clear, between how people define their self-worth and controlling their eating habits and spoke about the reciprocal relationship between the female body and what a woman allows it to receive based on her conscious and unconscious beliefs about what she deserves. In Orbach;s book, which was part critical essay, part guide, she tried to look at a woman's weight gain as an intentional affront, conscious and unconscious, against the restrictions of gender roles as they are defined in our culture.

A little under twenty years later, Naomi Wolf, one of the leaders of the third wave of American feminism, also took on the perception of women's bodies from a social-political standpoint in her resounding book *The Beauty Myth*. She claims slimness has become a tool for the oppression of women who erase themselves in their attempt to achieve it.

Susan Bordo, another feminist researcher and part of the post-modernist movement, claims the body functions as a cultural text, and as a direct focus of social control. She talks about the female body as something women submissively put a lot time into managing and disciplining using discipline that has become routine like dieting, makeup, and dressing, women have become focused on self-repair. Bordo sees the female body as an arena of struggle, of resisting gender superiority, and not serving gender normalization and submission.

Following these leading writers, the feminist discourse about female fat continued examining the question: how should we understand the bodies of fat women? Is it possible that the fat body expresses a renunciation of the need to conform to the demands from it as a feminine body? Is it possible that a woman who refuses to take part in dieting and the pursuit of for thinness is in many ways a woman who dares to free herself from oppressive social duress?

Towards the end of the 20th century and the beginning of the 21st century, the discussion about the body embraced a wide social context, including both the masculine and the feminine. Today there is an agreement that obesity should not be looked at as the problem of a specific minority and is difficult to ascribe to a certain age, gender, sexual orientation, or race. "The body is a site on which regimes of discourse and power inscribe themselves, a nodal point or nexus for relations of juridical and productive power," said Foucault[3]. It is the site of the greatest struggle in human history. A struggle between oppressive social forces on one hand and the self-perception of the individual.

In the last decade we witnessed the rise of a new cultural and political discourse titled "Fat Studies." This discourse came about due to the movement for the acceptance of people who had different body sizes. This movement, tries to promote the equality of human rights and speak against the connection made between a person's weight and his identity and value. Both in his own eyes and those of society. They try to break the link between excess body weight and obesity and an etiology of illness and mortality, lack of aesthetic, moral, and character flaws, negligence, and low socio-economic status. This struggle is growing along with weight discrimination, which is perceived as "the new homophobia," or "fatophobia." In the first decade of the 21st century, a number of studies showed a 66% increase in the occurrence of weight discrimination.

Facts began to come to light which revealed that for most people, dieting is a legacy of failure. This didn't stop the diet industry from continuing to make unprecedented efforts to "help" people lose weight. Dieting has recently become the most successful failure in the modern age, which creates revenue of over 60 billion dollars a year in the UnitedStates alone.

For nearly 15 years I have been an active member in the diet industry. The realization that I am not helping my patients, and even harming them by attempting to help them lose weight, was a point of no return for me. I realized that the playing field was different from what I thought it to be. I also realized the global obesity epidemic is controlled by powerful political and economic forces. I saw that the all-encompassing "truth" about the dangers of weight gain was not as it was presented to be. This does not mean "let's be fat", but it also doesn't mean that we have to be thin in order to be healthy, and there are situations in which extra weight can act as a protective agent. I also discovered that the attempt to lose weight itself causes weight gain and many harmful problems, some obvious, some hidden. The eating habits of many people has been disrupted. It drifts from dieting to binging. We have lost our natural codes of hunger and satiation and in many cases lost the pleasure and joy of food as well. Eating that was meant to be natural and intuitive has become eating ruled by laws. The person's relationship with his body has been damaged and weight set as his status as what defines our self-identity.

I began asking questions:

- Why does a person who loses weight gain it back?
- Is weight really a result of will power?
- Is obesity the result of a caloric equation?
- Is body weight a correct gauge of health?
- What is the damage caused to a person when he is part of the gain weight-lose weight cycles?
- Is it possible that as a therapist I am unintentionally harming my patients, reinforcing and perpetuating their weight problem?

Step by step, without first considering it, I began leading my patients in another direction. I felt in a very real, though painful, way, that I was no longer able to "sell the thin dream." I resigned from my position as the head of the Israeli Dietician Association so I could act in an interest free manner, in accordance with my heart's faith and my professional integrity. This wasn't easy. The patients continued chasing the magic cure-all that would allow them to achieve their dreams of becoming thin. They were willing to pay a fortune in order to achieve it. And I, as a professional who didn't believe in and was not willing to sell dreams, began losing patients and money and earning endless criticisms. It was hard and painful. But there was no turning back.

Today I try to help people free themselves from their pursuit of weight loss, and help them realize that it is possible to live without numbers on the scale running their lives. I work from a world view based on health focused approaches which have earned the nickname "HAES"- Health at Every Shape and Size. At their foundation is the recognition that there is now no sustainable solution to obesity and that 95% of those who lose weight gain it back within five years. They assume that the strive for thinness does not lead people to health and a full life, while eating with mindfulness to natural codes of hunger and satiation can led anyone to the body weight that's right for them. A weight that does not necessarily match the social model of beauty or BMI measurements. These approaches also believe that health is not measured in pounds and the dangers lurking in extreme weights do not apply to the majority of the population. The objective is not to create a thin human race, but healthy lives for people of all shapes and sizes.

This new, nonconformist path of mine is a difficult one. In order to walk it, I have enlisted theories from the world of nonjudgmental, mindfulness based advanced behavioristic cognitive therapy. Its roots are in Buddhism, and its arrival in the western world can be accredited to Jon Kabat-Zinn. These therapeutic approaches draw their ideological basis from eastern philosophies, from existential theories, and from cognitive behavioral theories.

At the heart of the matter I will present- as a metaphor, and a source of inspiration- the four noble truths that are the foundations of Buddhism:

Dukkah: The truth of the existence of suffering.Life in the world is not satisfying, not harmonious, and includes suffering. Suffering is universal.

Smodia: The truth of the origin of suffering.There is a simple reason for suffering-ignorance.

Nirvana: The truth of the expulsion of suffering.It is possible to free oneself from ignorance and thus free oneself from suffering. Suffering is not inevitable.

Marga: the truth of the path to freedom from suffering. There is a path that leads to the end of suffering.

Think about these truths in regards to weight gain and the suffering involved in dissatisfaction with our bodies and accept the foundations of the approach laid before you:

- Weight gain and the suffering it entails is universal.
- The dream of thinness and the Diet Language causes this suffering.
- It is possible to free oneself from the grasp of the thin dream and the Diet Language.
- Mindful Eating is the path to release.

The book does not stick to one approach. Rather, it creates a unique therapeutic, ideological mix which will best serve the process of separation from the dieting trap to replace it with a new language, one of Mindful Eating, which will lead us to living a full and healthy life with the body weight each and every one of us was meant to be.

Whenever I think about society's difficulty to accept this new approach, Wislawa Szymborska's[4] beautiful words come to mind in the parable of the fishermen and the letter:

"Some fishermen pulled a bottle from the deep. In it was a scrap of paper, on which were written the words: "Someone, save me! Here I am. The ocean hascast me up on a desert island. I am standing on the shore waiting for help.

Hurry. Here I am"!

"There is no date. Surely it is too late by now. The bottle could have been floating in the sea a long time," said the first fisherman.

"And the place is not indicated. We do not even know which ocean," said the second fisherman.

"It is neither too late nor too far. The island called Here is everywhere," said the third fisherman.

They all felt uneasy. A silence fell. So it is with universal truths."

PART ONE: THE DIET LANGUAGE CAUSES SUFFERING

King William the Conqueror won the Battle of Hastings in 1066, but when the battle was over he was unable to mount his horse because he was too fat. This shame brought the English king to a revolutionary decision, an unprecedented one: from now he will be on a strict diet. He must lose weight. A king who cannot mount his horse is unworthy of a crown.

William the Conqueror chose a unique diet: he replaced solid food with large quantities of wine. But to his surprise the dietary change did not help. The king rarely left his bed and ballooned to alarming proportions. He gained many pounds and eventually died after falling off of a horse and rupturing his stomach. William the Conqueror's attempt in the 11th century is considered the first documented case of a person taking pronounced measures to shed excess fat- and failing.

Obesity is a disease and weight loss is the solution. That is the common belief. Studies have since refuted this assumption, and from my experience I have learned that it is far from reality, but even so, this is still the given opinion among the masses. Continue on to the next chapters- the point of this book- which deal with the ways to be freed from this concept and the suffering it causes.

We should take another moment to consider a fundamental question: what is obesity?

The accepted global method for gauging obesity is the Body Mass Index(BMI) weight in kilograms divided by height in meters squared. This method was suggested by the Belgian statistician and mathematician Adolph Quetelet in 1830 as a means of classifying the population and not as a tool to predict health or mortality. About one hundred and forty years later, in 1972, the American nutritionist and epidemiologist Ancel Keys gave the system its name- the BMI scale, and used it to gauge excess weight. According to this scale, adults suffering from grade one obesity are those with a BMI grade higher than 30 and lower than 34.9.

Since the beginning of the twenty first century, substantial scientific evidence has been gathered stating that "weight gain" in its problematic sense is not a disease of pounds, as we mistakenly thought, and as the BMI* indicates, but it is a symptom of fat cells not functioning. Obesity is a metabolic and genetic issue. In metabolic terms, between twenty and thirty percent of those defined "overweight are healthy and between twenty and thirty percent of those defined "thin" are unhealthy.

Therefore, weight is not a single and satisfactory sign of sickness or health.

THE OBESITY SYNDROME

Obesity in its problematic sense will be defined in the book before you as a complex syndrome, at the center of which are skewed metabolic patterns. The severity of the problem can be gauged using four measures:

- An abnormal metabolic profile (blood lipids, blood sugar levels, blood pressure).
- Height to weight ratio according to the BMI scale.
- Functional limitations - physical, social, professional, emotional - that are attributed to body weight.
- The individual's personal experience when bearing all of the labels attached to the term "obese person", including lack of will power, laziness, and loss of value and identity.

In this book the definition for those who have the

---

* The BMI scale is a controversial measure and is used in this text only because there is no other scientifically proven measure.

obesity syndrome will be those for whom at least two of these four measures exist.

The traditional definition of obesity fits in with the mechanistic philosophy, which regards good health as the absence of risk factors. According to this outlook, obesity is a disease and health is the lack of disease. The weight centered approach assumes that losing weight is essential to improving health. The way to do this, according to the U.S. Centers for Disease Control and Prevention (CDC), is by making a lifestyle change and increasing physical activity. The primary premise at the root of this perception is that losing weight is the result of will power, thus any person is able to lose weight and reach his target goal, as stipulated by the BMI scale.

By this approach, any and all means should be taken to lose weight, and the consensus about the most efficient ways to lose weight changes with what is in vogue.. The diet culture that ruled the arena up to the first decade of the 21st century which included mainly caloric indication, nutritional guidelines, and specific menus, has been replaced by a new concept: "A Lifestyle Change." This change includes giving nutritional information like calorie counting, fat percentages, food substitutes and labels, social support, physical activity to improve health and maintain weight and use of behavior changing techniques (control techniques, positive reinforcements) in peoples' efforts to lose weight.

Most of the lifestyle change techniques offer behavioral methods to reduce consumption and guidelines for removal or restriction of certain foods that are labeled as unhealthy and fattening. The main objective is nutritious, low calorie eating, which along with physical activity will enable weight loss. In recent years this term has caught on and is now the accepted message in the war on fat. In many ways this is the same as the twentieth century "diet", but under a different title.

> *A diet is any eating program or procedure whose objective, whether overtly or covertly, is weight loss*

This is also the non-diet approach, another trendy new method joining its predecessors. Non-diet equals losing weight without going on a diet. The objective: to lose weight by dealing with emotional eating and misconceptions developed about food and eating which are getting in the way of achieving the desired weight. An array of different techniques like psychodrama, behavioral cognitive therapy, NLP, theta healing, and personal coaching are also involved in the weight loss crusade.

It is interesting to see how strong, influential, and vast these trends are, even though it has since been proven that the quest for losing weight is destined to fail: 95% of people who lose weight gain it back within one to five years, which is a cause of ongoing suffering for many. [5,6,7]

> *A diet- any diet, even a disguised one- is a legacy of failure for 95% of people*

JUST TO LOSE WEIGHT

The internet is bursting with promises. Everyone's selling thinness by marketing it wrapped in colorful ribbons and sounds of magical happiness awaiting whoever can make it through. And who'll give up?

This was how the parents of a 12 year old girl from a small town in southern Israel reached me. I hoped that the tyranny of thinness had missed them. It seemed as if this was their problem rather than the little girl's. Their daughter is a beloved good sport, and a good student. It's true that she sometimes gets a snide comment from some kid or other, but she has the inner strength to not let this get in her way. But they don't. To be exact, the mother, who had just lost 16 pounds and was battling their automatic rise back, doesn't. And she hops from liposuction to slimming treatments to acupuncture, works out four times a week, and this child of hers gives her away. She's a painful testament of what she used to be and what she can't imagine being again.

She pays a severe cost, but it seems to me that no price can be put on her difficulty to love her daughter. Her inability to touch her, to hug her, to smile at her, to take pride in her. And she does not let go, always trying to change her child like she does herself. Berating her. Over-controlling what she eats. Shooting her scornful glances. And I was innocently convinced that she was coming to me so I'd help her not to hurt her daughter, but to my shock I discovered that her only wish is to get her rebellious daughter thin. To get her to fit in with the thinness ideal.

THE OBESITY PARADOX

These fads- diets, lifestyle change, Non diet approach- are based on a variety of myths that have become deeply rooted in the human experience, and they are difficult to uproot. Myths which are at the forefront of the intimidation campaign against weight gain and the incredible desire to lose weight at any cost. According to them:

- Over weight and obesity lead to premature mortality
- Overweight and obesity lead to morbidity
- Weight loss is the way to ensure health and longevity

"More and more studies point to the possibility that excess weight does not necessarily shorten life expectancy. But many health researchers are refusing to acknowledge this." This is the opening statement of an article published in *Nature*[8] in May, 2013. It marked the end of acting as the resonating final chord of a raging debate which took place following the publication of a study by one of the leading researchers in the U.S's CDC, Prof. Kathryn Flegel, in the January 2003 issue of the famous *JAMA*[9]publication. The study, led by Dr. Flegel, surveyed 97 studies held in 12 countries around the world and included about 3 million participants. It tested the risk of mortality in normal weight and in the different levels of obesity as defined by BMI measures. The findings showed that in comparison to people of normal weight, those that were overweight (*30*>BMI>25) were 6% less at risk of mortality, and those in grade 1 obesity(30<BMI<35) were 5% less at risk.

Prof. Flegel[10] dared to present these revolutionary findings in 2005. Even then her study took the medical world by storm and even then she confronted prominent members of the medical establishment who treated every person with a bit of fat on them as if he were ill and destined for premature mortality. She demonstrated that the lower concentration of mortality risk factors were actually found in those with overweight (BMI 25-30), while moderate obesity (BMI 30-35) did not cause a higher risk than with normal weight. The study's conclusion was that extreme over weight (morbid obesity) is indeed dangerous to health, but a few extra pounds may actually reduce mortality risks. The researchers conjectured that the risk of test subjects who have reasonable over weight and ate healthily and regularly exercised, was lower in comparison to those defined as being of normal body weight. Those at the edges- very thin or very fat- are at the highest risk of mortality.

> *Extreme obesity is dangerous to health, as is extreme underweight, but it is possible that a few extra pounds actually reduces mortality risks*

In September 2012, a follow up study was published in the *European Heart Journal*[11] that spanned over three years and took place in Sweden. The study demonstrated that those who underwent a catheterization and were with obesity by BMI standards had a lower risk of mortality than those who have normal body weight or have underweight. Dr. Kristjan Karason, one of those conducting the study, further added that it is unclear why, but obesity may even act as a certain protective factor for people with chronic cardiac disease. Dr. Stefhan D. Anker, Dr. Oliver Hartman, and Dr. Stefhan Von Haelin, senior researchers from the Charite' School of Medicine in Germany, reinforce these findings and say: "Weight loss among people with chronic morbidity and with a BMI of under 40 may be a bad thing."

The term "obesity paradox" was first used officially in 2002 by Gruberg[12] and his research associates who wished to describe the unexpected results that emerged from their study. The results showed that overweight and obese people with coronary artery disease who underwent a catheterization had better results in the short and long term. They suffered from less complications in hospitalization and less cardiac mortality than normal weight or underweight people. Obesity paradox perfectly describes the latest findings, demonstrating that excess weight may increase the risk of heart disease, cancer, and other chronic illnesses, but for some people, especially middle aged and older, some extra weight was found to be not necessarily harmful and even possibly helpful and efficient. It is important to note that "extremely overweight", that is especially "fat" (BMI < 35), will nearly always be dangerous to health.

A study published that year in the *New England Journal of Medicine*[13], a renowned professional publication, examined the link between BMI and the incidence of heart failure in nearly 5900 participants in the Framingham study. During 14 years of tracking, it was foreseen that any rise in BMI category increased the risk of heart failure by 46% in women and 37% in men. It was also foreseen that in comparison to a normal BMI, participants with a tendency to overweight (BMI over 30) would have double the risk of heart failure (a 112% increased risk for women and 90% for men). But when they attempted to examine the connection between body weight and morbidity and mortality from heart disease in patients who already had heart disease, they paradoxically found an inverse link between obesity and cardiovascular morbidity and mortality. Dr. Carl Lavie, the Medical Director of the Cardiac Rehabilitation and Preventive Cardiology Department at the John Ochsner Hospital in New Orleans, was one of the first researchers to document this paradox in patients with heart failure as early as 2002. He spent over a year attempting to publish his findings in a journal, since no one actually believed his findings were correct.

The diabetes researcher Mercedes Carenthon, from Northwestern University, also mulled over the conundrum.If obesity is a principal risk factor for type 2 diabetes, why do a significant number of people with normal body weight develop this disease? In her study, she discovered that diabetics with normal weight had double the risk of dying than diabetics with overweight or with obesity.

A meta-analysis[14] from 2008 analyzed data from nine studies held among 28,209 people with chronic heart disease. The tracking period was 2.7 years on average. The findings showed that in patients with overweight (BMI 25-30) there was a 16% lower rate of overall mortality and 19% lower rate of cardiovascular mortality while in patients with obesity (BMI over 30) the corresponding differences were 33% in overall mortality and 40% in cardiovascular mortality. When a standardized analysis was done, it was still found that the risk of mortality in being overweight or obese is lower. It is interesting to note that in none of the nine studies included in the analysis was there even one study that demonstrated a reduced risk of mortality in people with normal weight or were with underweight in comparison to people with overweight or with obesity.

An additional study published in 2007[15] examined the link between BMI and the mortality risk in acute coronary disease. The study was held in 263 hospitals in the U.S. and included 108,927 patients overall who were admitted for acute heart failure. The study discovered that mortality rates in admission were linked inversely to BMI.

Benderly and Goldbourt[16] examined the link between relative weight among 12,466 Israeli cardiac patients (most of them with a history of myocardial infarction) throughout 12 years. The "normal weight" subjects whose BMI was 20-23 showed mortality rates that were not significantly smaller than those in the 23-30 range. Professor Goldbourt, a researcher of epidemiology and preventative medicine at Tel Aviv University, says, "In the not-so-old school, it was recommended to supposedly 'overweight' cardiac patients (BMI 25-30) to lose weight. This recommendation must become a thing of the past, because it dangerously contradicts the results of a series of epidemiologic studies published in recent years."

The issue of body weight is tightly linked to physical fitness. In the past it was believed that physical fitness has a principal role in the weight loss process, but as it has been realized that dieting is a legacy of failure, it has also been realized that the benefits of physical fitness to the weight loss process is questionable. However, in the last decade it has become clear that physical fitness has an essential role in sustaining our health, maybe even a bigger role than body weight.

In a study held by the Longevity Institute in the Cooper Instituteof preventive medicine, data from over [17] 34,000 men and women was gathered. The study's results proved that the mortality rates were lower when the fitness level was higher, with no connection to body weight. In other words, a person of above average weight who is in good shape has a better chance of longevity than a thin person who sits in front of the TV all day. The important input to our discussion on the issue of weight is that weight loss has not been found to increase chances of quality of life and longevity.

An additional study[18] was held at the Cooper Institute of Aerobics, examining the link between physical activity and the risk of mortality over eight and a half years in 25,389 men, some with normal weight and some with overweight. The study's findings clearly showed that poor physical fitness is more dangerous than obesity.

The effect of physical training on women with obesity (with a BMI of 35) and its effect on women with normal weight (BMI=21) who lead a "sedentary" lifestyle was examined over 14 weeks[19]. Each group consisted of 40 participants whose average age was forty eight. The study's results proved that the two groups improved their physical fitness (cardiovascular system and aerobic fitness) at a similar rate, with no change in weight. The researchers' conclusion was that it was not necessary to lose weight in order to improve physical fitness.

A four year tracking of the health of 906 women[20] whose average age was fifty eight and 76% of them with a BMI over 25, showed that a lack of physical activity is a bigger risk factor for developing heart disease than a BMI of 25. It is possible, then, to say that long term health is dependent on physical activity.

One of the senior researchers in the U.S. CDC, Professor Kathryn Flegel, stated simply: "The link between mortality and lack of physical fitness is much stronger than the link between mortality and obesity."

An additional study supporting this evidence, held in 13,155 men with high blood pressure and published in 2009[21], found a strong inverse link between physical fitness and mortality in the obese participants. Meaning among men with high blood pressure who were in good physical shape, there was no increase in risk of heart disease or any other mortality risk factor.

> *Fat and fit is healthier than thin and not fit*

You can say, then, that people with obesity according to the Body Mass Index, who are physically fit, are not at greater risk of cardiac morbidity in comparison to people with normal weight, by that same measure, who are physically fit. Furthermore, people with obesity in good shape are at less of a risk in comparison to people with normal weight whose physical fitness is lacking. So as it turns out, physical activity is a significant long-term relative advantage for all people, in all shapes and sizes.

These findings and their likes require an explanation. In addition to the BMI scale being a problematic health assessment tool, many studies presumed that the risk of cardio-metabolic morbidity and diabetes doesn't have to do with how much fat is accumulated in the body overall, but more with how fat is distributed in the different tissues and the function of fat cells in them. Also, it is possible that many studies which formed the connection between obesity and mortality suffered from a wrong translation of the results resulting from different deviations in the study population. It is also possible that the population suffering from obesity and comorbidity is better treated and therefore diagnosis of the illness and treatment of it is earlier and allows tracking that may cause a decrease in morbidity and mortality.

Other explanations which have been suggested are that people with overweight get a relative advantage since their heart does more work. This work is a factor of weight multiplied by distance. For example, at the same distance, people of a higher weight exert more physical effort than people of a low weight.

The existence of the obesity paradox is no longer questionable, though the mechanism at its root is still unclear. We can summarize by saying that today four paradoxes exist that are related to obesity[22].

- **Classic obesity paradox**- Assumes that there are cases in which obesity is a protective factor against chronic diseases, like heart disease, especially in older age.

- **Pre-obesity paradox**- Assumes that excess weight acts as a protective factor in the regular and normal population.

- **The fat and fit paradox**- Assumes that when people are physically fit, their body weight does not cause an increased risk of mortality.

- **The healthy fat paradox**- Claims some adults with obesity have a sound cardio-metabolic profile. Findings show that 30% of people with first degree obesity are as metabolically healthy as thin people.

Dr. Dror Dicker, Head of Internal Medicine D and the Clinic for Obesity and Hypertension at Rabin Medical Center, sums up the issue by saying "Obesity is not a disease of kilograms, it is a disease of malfunctioning fat cells." According to him, "Many findings demonstrate lack of connection between weight or BMI and longevity and improvement in morbidity or mortality. The understanding today is that the function of fat cells is what's responsible for a person's metabolic health. If a fat cell can expand and grow enough while supplying the proper amount of blood to the body, the person will be metabolically healthy even in situations of caloric excess, but if the fat cells are unable to expand and grow in a satisfactory manner in caloric excess or the blood flow does not correspond with growing fat tissue, due to a genetic reason or an apparent environmental reason (like smoking), the fatty tissue will undergo processes of necrosis (gangrene), inflammation and cellular breakdown while creating a widespread inflammatory process and surfacing free fatty acids which sink into organs like the liver and pancreas, muscle and the heart, creating for instance, a resistance to insulin, diabetes and metabolic morbidity. This situation can occur in extreme thinness or any thinness due to malfunction of fat tissue and cells and create a situation of thin metabolic illness. This understanding disconnects the responsibility for metabolic and cardiovascular morbidity from weight, transferring this responsibility to the function of fat cells."

> *Obesity is not a disease of kilograms but of malfunctioning fat cells*

Even so, caution is advised when making sweeping conclusions when it comes to obesity as a risk factor for morbidity and mortality. These findings shed a different light on many beliefs and perceptions about the dangers of obesity that are not necessarily based on evidence. They raise questions like, is there a justified basis for all encompassing recommendations to lose weight for those with a BMI of over 25? Is it possible that a few extra pounds may actually increase life span?

The sweeping approach which assumes obesity is necessarily harmful and causes increased morbidity and mortality should undergo some sort of renewal and reexamination, and every individual person and his metabolic measures should be considered. After all, the realization is beginning to seep in with the establishment-you don't have to be thin to be healthy.

Even the U.S. CDC dropped obesity from second to seventh place in the global ranking of mortality risks in 2005. But the intimidation campaign against obesity continues.

> *Weight is not a measure of health*

WEIGHT IS EVERYTHING

"You have to lose weight. Have to," the family doctor told her. "The pain in your knees is only from your extra weight. It's useless to send you to any further examination until you lose a few kilograms. Come back in a month after you've lost about 4 kilos and we'll see."

She was shocked. At a loss for words. He really can't see she's suffering? What does he think, that she's making it up? She's sick of the fact that everywhere, every sensation she has is linked to her weight. Society tells her, "If you lose weight you'll have a boyfriend, your back won't hurt, your stomach won't give you trouble, you won't have any headaches. One medicine can cure it all." And she? She tried it all. Lost it and gained it over and over again. What did they want from her?"

She left his office feeling crushed, dragging her leg as she walked. For two months she hasn't done any physical activity, she just can't. The family doctor disregards her, the orthopedic she turned to also refuses to take her seriously. She feels rejected. Lonely.

She's sitting in front of me. What can I say to her? How will I protect her? I, who knows her struggle with weight. Who knows her insecurity, the anger suffocating her, anger at this world which refuses to see her as a whole person, with feelings, abilities, needs and aches.

This is how she grew up. She was always led to believe she's no more than "weight". That she is "kilograms". , And she is always busy proving that she's worthy and equal. But nobody sees, nobody acknowledges her value. She is trapped in her own body, despising every single part of it. Fighting an eternal battle with this existence.

And then she comes to this doctor who also sees only weight. Who also refuses to see beyond this measure of kilograms she weighs and binds everything with her body weight, leaving her helpless. Despondent.

UNDERSTANDING THE PURSUIT OF THINNESS

"The real world doesn't take flight
the way dreams do.
No muffled voice, no doorbell
can dispel it,
no shriek, no crash
can cut it short.
Images in dreams
are hazy and ambiguous,
and can generally be explained
in many different ways.
Reality means reality:
that's a tougher nut to crack."[23]

Now it is clear that the worship of thinness is not based on healthy logic. And it is clear that the intimidation campaign against obesity is not anchored in reality and reason. It is also clear that the fear of gaining weight and our constant need to lose weight causes suffering. I will now invite you to stop for a moment and look at the way we hold on to the pursuit of thinness. Pause for a moment on the manner in which we grasp onto a thought and behavior pattern which hurts us on several levels and in many aspects.

Thinness was not always the beauty ideal. In 1825 a French author named Jean Anthekme Brillant-Sava wrote, "Thinness is a horrible thing for a woman. No matter how beautiful she is, something from her feminine mystique will be lost." Who would write such things today?

Much has been written about the beauty ideal and the thinness ideal. I will not attempt to delve into investigating this phenomenon, but focus my gaze on the relentless hold it has on us. We hold on to the thinness ideal as if we're holding on to a sinking boat. We know it's sinking, but we're afraid to let go. And how could we? We who are susceptible to the anti-fat intimidation campaign calling day in and day out: "A nation in danger." "Today's children are the first generation whose lives will be shorter than their parents' lives." "The obesity epidemic." "One out of every four children is fat." "If child obesity continues it will cut off between 2-5 years from their lives." "Junk food is dangerous." "Only one piece of candy a day." "Be careful of sugary drinks." "Fat kids-fat adults." "War on weight."

Alongside this, taxes on fattening foods, calorie labels in restaurants, weighing laws and weigh in cards for school children, laws against vending machines in schools, restrictions on commercials, harrowing statistics about morbidity and mortality rates associated with obesity, gym promotions touting the thin ideal… the list goes on. A perfect campaign. No one can stay indifferent to it.

And the grasp on the thinness ideal only becomes tighter. Whoever holds it is holding on to the perception that weight defines his identity, his value and his physical, emotional, moral and cognitive abilities. This grasp is perceived in our experience, in many ways, as one that saves lives. And giving it up is "death." If obesity has so many negative social and medical implications, who would want to be associated with it? What's developing here is a dangerous and violent anxiety: parents tyrannizing their children, couples berating one another and people hurting themselves.

In this context the interests of the diet industry, the fashion industry, and the plastic surgery industry are clear- as well as other businesses who make a profit of people's aversion to their bodies, whether male or female. What's relevant to us is to notice the way in which we ourselves hold on to the myth that has been dispelled and found to be harmful.

Our passion to be thin and our fear of gaining weight - our clinging to these harmful perceptions - creates suffering.

We are always craving something. A new friend,

delicious food, hungry for love, recognition, touch. There is almost never a moment in which we are not longing for something. There is almost never a moment when that craving is gone. We always want more. More money, more assets, more status, more love, more success. The feeling of "I don't have enough" reigns. Man does not exist without desire. It is what pushes him forward, to discover, to invent, to explore. But herein lies the catch. You cannot go through a whole life without experiencing pain, just as you cannot lead a whole life based on the Pleasure Principle alone. The strive for perfection will always be at the base of suffering. And its source is in the illusion that perfection is possible. As long as thinness will be labeled in our mind as the embodiment of happiness we persevere in chasing after it, and as long as obesity will be labeled as causing pain, we will steadfastly run away from it. In the space between them- we will go on suffering.

The data of the Central Bureau of Statistics from 2011 shows that over half of the population, 54 percent, want to lose weight: one third of those who have normal weight, 68 percent of those who have overweight and 88 percent of those who have obesity. In practice, about a fifth of the population is dieting; all the others are busy licking the wounds left by their former diets or searching for the next one to go on. There is nearly no person today who is not preoccupied with his weight and the need to change it in some way or other.

Diets, whether overt or covert, that emphasise "lifestyle change" or "non diet approch", lead at best to short-term weight loss- this loss is not sustained. In long-term studies it was found that for most of the population, adopting dietetic behaviors does not lead to weight loss or preservation, but actually triggers binge eating and weight gain. It seems that people who manage to lose weight and keep it off are the exceptional ones and that most people who lose weight, gain it back after some time. At times even more than what they'd lost.

In addition to weight loss failure, studies show that preoccupation with body weight disrupts eating, damages self-esteem, increases the incidence of eating disorders, and raises the weight gain bar. Furthermore, the younger the age in which preoccupation with weight begins, the higher the risk of weight gain, disruption of the child's healthy growing process, and disruption of his intuitive eating habits.

> *Preoccupation with body weight disrupts eating, damages self-esteem, increases the incidence of eating disorders, and causes obesity*

HAVE TO LOSE IT

"It's all because of my weight. I'm depressed because of it. I don't work and don't create. I'm at home because of it. With no friends, and of course with no girlfriend. I have to lose weight," he said "Have to. Only then will I be able to move forward with my life. That's what's blocking me."

He looked at me, staring. Convinced the thoughts running his life are true, convinced the world is measured entirely by those kilograms, which allegedly define his worth. And he eats. Without really noticing taste, hunger, or satiation. Why should he? All is lost. Until he loses weight there is no point to his life. Weight is everything. Success, happiness, health. The absurd thing is that he recently ran some blood tests and everything was normal. "But who cares," he said, "now I'm depressed and I have to lose weight." And I sit before him, as if my hands were cuffed. Knowing no diet will do him any good. Also knowing that the belief he holds that when he loses weight his troubles will disappear is also fundamentally mistaken. My sense of helplessness cries out deep inside, disturbing my self-confidence. And there are no tricks up my sleeve. He's dead set on his goal so much, surgery would seem like a diet to him. He'll shed dozens of kilos and gain them back. And then?

I try to explain. Talk about the Diet Language. About the way it warps eating. Explain to him that it was what was causing him to lose control of his eating and eat food that seems unhealthy. I talk about changing his perception and language. About listening to the body. About the process. But he sticks to his guns. He has to lose weight right now. And I look at him. At the kilograms padding his body. He pursues his goal with a stubbornness that won't let go of the misconception that weight is the measure for everything in life. I know that by doing this he continues to do more of the same. Perpetuating his situation, not creating a new horizon.

THE BODY RESISTING CHANGE

THE BODY PRESERVES ITS WEIGHT

The body is a control system, regulating food consumption and energy exertion, so weight and body composition- fat, proteins and liquids- are usually kept stable in adult life. Each and every person's body weight is set in part by a hereditary trait in the hypothalamus in the brain. Changes in body weight above or below the point of individual set-point stimulate the central nervous system to activate appetite and metabolism in order to protect that set-point. Every person has a group of set-points specific to him, that does not necessarily reflect the ideal weight as defined by BMI measures. Usually, a drop of 5 to 10 percent in body weight is enough to reach the set-point. It is possible to stabilize at that point by healthy eating, based on minding codes of hunger and satiation, without the sense of restriction, guilt or avoidance, along with physical activity.

It is important to state that it is easy to gain weight above the set point, but harder to lose it. The yo-yo effect of dieting causes the set-point to always be on the rise.

> *Every person has a set-point which is his destined weight*

Imagine for example a "Roly Poly" toy. When it's not touched it balances on a certain median, lightly wobbling over it. If you tilt it and press hard it will stay down until you let go.The harder the tilt, the more trouble it will have to stop at the initial median and will move a bit to the side. Our body is the same. When we're on a diet and push ourselves to enforce its rules, we stay at a low body weight as long as we succeed in avoiding temptations, and follow the rules. But one little mistake, one covert little slip up and the body "runs away." The binges and the uncontrolled eating begin. And body weight slowly returns to what it was before the diet. Sometimes when the weight loss is extreme, a slight increase in weight can occur until it gets higher than the starting point before the diet.

POST DIET

Abolishing the sensation of hunger by different limitations and diversions is probably the main cause of the failure of long-term diets. While in the short-term weight loss increases sensitivity to leptin (the hormone responsible for regulating appetite), improves tolerance for glucose (a monosaccharide) and reduces triglycerides, in the long-term, studies do not support ignoring homeostatic signals (which maintain the balance and stability of the body's internal environment when the external environment changes) for hunger and satiation. It seems that even a small nutritional deficiency, stemming from a diet, restriction or avoidance is enough to make the body feel threatened and provoke systems that work to correct the deficit by secreting hormones which increase hunger.

Evidence of this can be found in recent studies showing that weight loss puts the body in a unique metabolic state, a sort of post-diet syndrome, distinguishing those who dieted and those who didn't try to lose weight in the first place. Studies also show that a full year after significant weight loss, people remain in what can be defined as a different biological state. Their body behaves as if it's starving, and works overtime to regain the lost kilograms. This defense mechanism includes a rise in the level of the gherlin hormone, also called the hunger hormone, a drop in the level of leptin, a hormone which suppresses appetite and increases the rate of metabolism, and a drop in the levels of a hormone called peptide YY which is also related to appetite suppression[24, 25].

These findings, even if they are not substantial enough, challenge traditional thought that sees weight loss as a combination of will power, determination, eating less, and exercising more. Even if the instructions to eat healthy and live an active life have merit, they don't take into account the fact that the body is fighting against the weight loss long after the diet is over.

Leibel and his colleague Michael Rosenbaum were pioneers in discovering a substantial part of what we know about how the body reacts to weight loss. Over 25 years they meticulously tracked one hundred and thirty people for periods of six months or more. The test subjects were housed in their research clinic, where every aspect of their body was measured. They started with a liquid diet of 800 calories a day, until they lost 10 percent of their body weight. After they reached this goal, they underwent a further series of examinations, while trying to sustain their new weight. The results showed that when persons lose 10 percent of their body weight, their metabolism is different than that of persons of similar proportions whose body weight is the same naturally.[26]

The study showed that following weight loss several changes take place, which translate to the body needing 250 to 400 less calories. For example, a woman who entered their study weighing 104 kilograms ate about 3,000 calories to maintain her weight.

After she dropped to 86 kilograms (that is, lost 17% of her body weight), they found she only needed 2,300 calories a day to maintain her new weight. This may sound like a lot, but compared to the woman who dieted and lost weight, a woman of similar measures who did not lose weight can consume 2,600 calories a day and still maintain her weight. That's 300 more calories than the woman who lost weight to get there[27].

Scientists are still trying to understand why the body

that has lost weight behaves so differently than a body of similar proportions that hasn't lost weight. Muscle biopsies that were taken before, during, and after the weight loss show that when we lose weight, muscle fibers change and they become more similar to "slow fibers" which are far more efficient. As a result of this, after weight loss, muscles burn 20%-25% less calories during everyday activities and moderate aerobic training than a person who is that weight naturally. The meaning is that people on a diet, who think they're burning 200 calories in a half hour power walk, are probably only exerting about 150 calories.

Another way in which the body fights weight loss is in changing the way the brain reacts to food. Rosenbaum and his colleague Joy Hirsch, a brain researcher, used a functional Magnetic Resonance Imaging (fMRI) scan in order to track patterns in the brains of people before and after weight loss. They watched them while they were looking at objects like grapes, gummy bears, chocolate, broccoli, cellular phones, and a yo-yo. After the weight loss, when the subject was seeing the food, the scans showed a stronger response in the areas of the brain connected to reward and a lower response in the areas connected to control. The findings showed that the body intensifies excitement from food and weakens will power and resistance against high calorie indulgences after the diet, in order to return to its weight prior to it. Rosenbaum said, "After we lose weight, the brain has a stronger emotional response to food. We want it more and the areas in the brain involved in restraint are less active. This, in addition to the body now burning fewer calories than expected, creates the perfect environment to regain the weight."

The length of time this state goes on in is unknown, but a primary study that was held at Columbia University suggests that the body may continue to defend its former weight as long as six years after weight loss. This does not mean that it is impossible to lose weight and keep it off, but only that it is extremely hard.

Over the years, more evidence has to light about not only how the body resists change, but that the use of diets in itself increases obesity and highly affects development of eating problems which may worsen and become eating disorders.

In one of the more well-known studies held in the U.S and led by Prof. Dianne Neumark[28], researchers tried to understand why dieting causes weight gain in the long run. The researchers' estimation was that a diet leads to taking on unhealthy habits such as reduced consumption of breakfast, reduced consumption of fruits and vegetables and less frequent physical activity. Habits that lead to weight gain in the long-term. Researchers found that over 56 percent of girls dieted (made a nutritional change in order to lose weight) at least once over the last year. This behavior was found to be linked with an increase in binge eating after five years. In addition, an interesting connection was found between dieting among girls and a decline in the frequency of eating breakfast and a decline in consumption of fruits and vegetables after five years. Among the boys, about one quarter reported dieting when the study began, and just like the girls, the study pointed to an increase in binge eating and a decrease in physical activity after five years.

A diet, in the conventional sense of the word, meaning a caloric and cognitive restriction, may cause increased physical, emotional, and cognitive hunger as well as binge eating. The restraint at its base is an effort of resistance and abstention, and those who forcefully restrain their eating are constantly worried about what they're eating, how much and when, for fear of gaining weight. They are also those who are prone to losing control over their eating and bingeing, more than those who don't experience prohibition or restriction. And to make things even more complicated and complex, any emotional event or change compelled the subjects to lose control.

Adolescents who reported dieting and preoccupation with weight loss were at twice the risk of being overweight five years later than adolescents who didn't report watching what they eat. This diet is one of the main reasons for weight gain after losing weight.

It is interesting to see that studies that examined babies found that if there is a mismatch between hunger and satiation signals transmitted by the child and the way the caretaker intercepts them and resolves them, this will cause an increase in the frequency of meals or the amount of food consumed, which will cause inadequate regulation in the baby and destroy his hunger and satiation system. This brings to an increase in energy consumption which leads to weight gain and obesity even in infancy.

As early as the 1990's, two Canadian researchers, Claude Bouchard and Angelo Tremblay, conducted a series of studies[29] in which they examined 31 pairs of male twins between the ages of 17 and 29 who sometimes overate and were sometimes on a diet. In one study, 12 pairs of twins were put under a 24 hour watch in college dormitories. Six days a week they ate 1,000 extra calories a day and on the seventh day they were allowed to eat normally. They could read, play video games or cards and watch television, but their workouts were limited to a 30 minute walk each day. During the 120 days of the study, the twins consumed 84 thousand calories beyond their basic needs. This binge should have come to a weight gain of about 11 kilograms (per calculation of 7,700 calories per kilogram). But some gained less than five kilos while others gained 13 kilos. The weight gained and the distribution of the excess fat in the body was almost identical between brothers, but between the different pairs of twins there were considerable differences.

For example, some of the twins accumulated three times more fat around their abdomen than the others. When the researchers conducted similar fitness studies with the twins, they discovered the same patterns inversely:

some of the twins lost more weight even though they maintained the same training regime. The findings, wrote the researchers, point to a certain "biological determinism" which makes a person more susceptible to gaining or losing weight.[30]

These findings send us back to 1962, when the thrifty gene hypothesis was first published. This gene, according to certain researchers, has an important role in sustaining fat mass in times of hardship and shortage.

THE GENETIC LOAD

Leafing through the pages of history reveals that in times of need, hunter-gatherers lived under a constant threat of actual starvation. The role of their genes responsible for the tendency for being overweight was essential, because they increased the energy reserves and provided a survivalist advantage in times of hunger. In comparison to the hunter-gatherers, people who descended from the Fertile Crescent area, who used to domesticate plants and animals, did not suffer from the dangers of starvation. According to the researchers, they may have less fattening, thrifty genes and more thin genes, adapted to an environment rich with food. This may tell us that people with overweight or obesity are those carrying the hunter-gatherer genes.

The body's ability to sustain the fat mass, which was meant to protect it in times of hunger, has become in our affluent society one of the causes of obesity. Proof of a significant genetic component in the obesity phenomenon can be found in the Native-American Pima tribe- a small ethnic group living by the Gila River in southern Arizona in the U.S. The tribe's people were diagnosed as the fattest people in the world. Over 75% of the tribes' population is defined obese, with a BMI of over 30. An average Pima male weighs 100 kilograms, and an average Pima female weighs 90.5 kilograms.

A person weighing 135 kilograms is not a rarity in the tribe. It seems the Pima gained weight due to the same reasons that cause obesity all around the western world: a diet high in fats and sugars and lack of physical activity. Until the second half of the twentieth century the Pima were lean and muscular due to an active lifestyle and a diet rich in fibers and low in sugars. With time the tribe embraced American lifestyle habits and gained weight. In comparison to the average American, this change was supposed to increase their weight by only a few kilos, but the Pima gained much more than a few kilos- this, many researchers claim, is due to the mutual influence of environment and genetics. Genes, as it were, do not necessarily make people fat, but they cause those with a tendency to gain weight to gain more weight because of the changing environment.

A reinforcement of this claim can be found in data from the World Health Organization in 2013 showing that although obesity is usually seen as a disease of the well fed, little moving western world, the rate of sufferers from overweight and obesity is actually highest in poor countries like the islands of American Samoa, the Kiribati islands, and the islands of French Polynesia. This data reinforces the genetic component in obesity. A new study from Ben Gurion University in association with Hadassah Medical Center in Jerusalem, also reinforces this complexity. The study, published in 2013, showed that the success of a diet does not depend solely on caloric intake or the type of food that is consumed, but also on our genetic load.

Genetics is a substantial component in the tendency for obesity. Dieting intensifies this tendency

---

While there is a widespread agreement that at least part

of the risk for obesity is hereditary, identifying the specific genetic factor has proven to be a challenge. In October 2010, *Nature Genetics*[31] reported that researchers have so far identified 32 genetic variances linked to obesity or BMI. One of the most common of them was identified in April 2007 by a British team investigating the genetics of diabetes. According to Timothy Frayling[32,33] from the Institute of Biomedical & Clinical Science at Exeter University, people with a variant called FTO are at a much higher risk of morbid obesity- 30% if they have one copy of the variant, 60% if they have two copies. This FTO variant is surprisingly common. The assumption is that about 65% of people of European or African descent and about 27% to 44% of Asians carry at least one copy of it. Scientists don't understand how the variant affects weight gain, but studies in children show it has a role in forming eating habits.[34,35]

In one study in 2008, led by Colin Palmer from Dundee University in Scotland, Scottish school children were given muffins and orange juice and were then offered a buffet that included grapes, celery, French fries, and chocolate which they were free to nibble from. The different types of food were meticulously supervised, so researchers knew exactly what was eaten. All of the children ate around the same amount of food, but kids with the FTO variant tended to prefer foods high in fat and calories. They didn't stuff themselves, but they consumed, on average, 100 calories more than the children without the gene. The carriers of the genetic variant had about two kilograms more body fat than the others.

THE MINNESOTA STUDY

The absurd thing is that the failure of the diet was clear even during World War Two, and this came to be seen in the well-known "Minnesota Study"[36] headed by Dr. Ancel

Keys. The study was done on a group of 36 healthy men with high psycho-biological durability. These were men who were completely free from concerns about their body weight and that prior to the experiment had never concerned themselves about the types and amounts of food they consumed. During the first three months of the experiment the participants consumed 3,492 calories a day. In the following six months their calorie consumption was reduced by 50% and was 1,570 calories a day (a half starvation ration). In addition to the fact that the participants in the study lost a quarter of their body weight, the experiment led to the following results: the participants' metabolism dropped by 40%, the participants' eating behaviors completely changed, some developed bulimia and most of them experienced uncontrolled eating and binges and once the study was over, found it difficult to return to their primary eating behaviors. They were preoccupied with what they were eating, how much and when, hung photos of desired foods over their beds, and after the war they chose professions that were somehow related to cooking. Some of them also experienced a change in personality like apathy, nervousness, restlessness, mood swings, and depression. The results of the study were far reaching, especially in light of the fact that the Minnesota Study was done before the era of thinness and diets, when the field of research in nutrition was still in its infancy. The researchers gathered from the study's results that not only does a diet provoke binge eating and excessive cognitive preoccupation with food, but that after a diet, the body is unable to sustain its new weight and strives to return to its primary weight.

A diet, any diet- is fattening

The National Weight Control Registry in the U.S follows 10,000 people who have lost weight and kept it off. The registry was founded as a point of proof against those who claim no one can lose weight and keep it off over time. In response to this, Prof. Kelly Brownell,[37] head of the Rudd Center for Food Policy and Obesity at the University of Connecticut, said that the 10,000 people tracked by the Registry are a helpful source of information, but represent a minute ammount of the tens of millions who have unsuccessfully attempted to lose weight. "The only meaning of this that there are some extraordinary individuals who succeed in maintaining their weight loss," said Brownell. "It turns out that these people are very strictly watching their weight. Years after the diet they still watch every calorie, exercise for an hour each day. They are always thinking about their weight."[38]

Dr. Albert J. Stunkard, one of the pioneers in the field of obesity research, said in 1959: "Most of the people who begin a weight loss program do not finish it, most of those who finish it do not lose weight, and most of the people who lose weight do not succeed in keeping it down."

DIETING - A FORETOLD FAILURE

"How old are you?" I asked. "Thirty six," she replied. "At what age did you go on your first diet and how much did you weigh then?" "I think I was 16 and a half and I weighed 65 kilos." "And today?" I asked further. "84 kilos," she replied, and her eyes began tearing up. Twenty years- twenty kilograms. And no, this was not her fault. Although she was convinced it was, despite the fact that she was able to list each of the dozens of diets she had been on throughout her life and described each and every diet to me with extreme detail, as well as the main reason for her gaining the weight back. The first one was because of her high school's final exams; the second one was right after the army because of a trip to the Far East. Two years later was a break up from a boyfriend, a big move...her list went on and on. Every event is a proven reason and justification for the failure of the diet. And of course she's the one to blame. She who has no spine or will power. She, who's convinced that cause for her failure lies at her door. She who swore to me that if I help her lose weight this time she definitely won't fail. She'll work hard, she said. She'll even go to the gym and stop buying potato chips.

THE DIET LANGUAGE- A LANGUAGE OF CONTROL

The need to lose weight and the belief that it is possible to lose weight by regulating caloric balance birthed various behavioral patterns, principally to do with control. Control over what you eat, how much, when and how, and control of how many calories you burn through physical activity. Diet is a regime. There are rules governing what is allowed and forbidden. There is enforcement- shame, guilt, or denunciation.

The pursuit of thinness, the diet that accompanies it, and the failure therein has created a language (for lack of a better term). A language of eating- the Diet Language. This is a language administrated by control, intimidation, abstention and threat and by an external imposition dictating what to eat, when, how much, how to feel and what to think before, during and after eating. This is a language nearly everyone speaks. It is spoken outside, in interpersonal communication, and spoken inside, in intrapersonal communication. We think, feel, and act according to this language which is:

A language of control, whose terms are materialistic and deterministic.A dichotomist language. In its terms, only what can be measured is real.

A language which doesn't do justice with our innate and intuitive ability as human beings, assuming that every person has natural codes of hunger and satiation.

A language which deprives us of the ability to know when and why we're hungry, when we're full, and from what foods.

A language which robs us of our free will, but mainly steals from us the joy of eating.

This is a language with its own vocabulary, including controlling, restricting, and intimidating words- allowed, forbidden, dangerous, unhealthy, healthy, limited, lazy, failed, fattening, non-fattening, starting tomorrow, just for today, if I'm doing it might as well, low, reduced, just today, just one...

- In the Diet Language we say things like these:
- You have to eat breakfast.
- I'll eat now and I won't eat later.
- Today I'll eat and starting tomorrow I'll watch it.
- I have to lose weight.
- I'm such a loser; I went off my diet again.
- I'm not going to the beach until I lose weight.
- Oh my god, I'm going on vacation tomorrow, what'll I do?
- Did you see the look of her?
- Why doesn't she do something with herself?
- Pizza is a dangerous food.
- Cake is a horrible, fattening thing.
- If you're fat, no one will want you.
- A fat person is lazy, and a loser.
- Eat now and abstain later.
- I'm not allowed to eat ice cream.
- I don't love myself.

Everyone speaks the Diet Language, which has also created social codes making it acceptable to invade one another's plate, to find out what they ate, how much and why. To comment about the size of their body. To whine about "I ate so much,"or "I've gained so much weight," and "I'm starting a diet tomorrow." No holds are barred. All borders are broken. Whoever isn't privy to this discourse finds themselves a bit excluded. Maybe even a little unequal. This language has created dress codes and codes of status. Social status is determined by weight. The lower it is- the higher your value. The Diet Language affects our state of mind, the way we're accepted in society, in the workplace, in the family, and our ability to enjoy our existence, with eating a central part of it.

This language led most of us to not only knowing what, how much, when, how and why to eat, but to our eating, which was meant to be intuitive and natural, became managed by a disorder. I won't be mistaken in saying that as a society we have an eating disorder. At the edges, we can place those suffering from eating disorders expressed by binge eating, self-induced vomiting, extreme thinness, and a warped body image on one end of the spectrum and those suffering from morbid obesity and the morbidity that accompanies it on the other. Although the statistics (according to the U.S. Academy of Eating Disorders) show that only 10% of the population are on those two ends of the spectrum, but in between them are the majority, who are not really "sick" in the common sense of the word but do suffer, on a daily basis, from a pained relationship with their body and eating. These people are the casualties of the use of the Diet Language.

> *The Diet Language is a language of control*

SHE'LL DO BETTER TOMORROW

The girls were sitting around the table in the local café. They were five. Soldiers on leave. They were holding the menu in their hands and giggling. They wore skinny jeans, tiny tee-shirts, and flats. The café was bustling, full of the sounds of rattling plates, chattering voices, and the scent of baking bread from the bakery next door. The menu lay before them and the usual discussion began. "Are we watching ourselves today?"

"Just a salad?"

"I have to watch myself today," one of them says, "I gained like two kilos this month."

The sun had left its peak, slowly sliding down. "Ugh, you and your salad," another whispers. "I'm sick of these diets."

"Easy for you to say, you're so skinny," the first one snaps. And the thin one, not one to be outdone, quickly replies, "Some good those diets are doing you...you're always suffering and pouting."

"Stop fighting," the one on the left says as she rushes to end the conversation. "We'll order some of everything," she decides.

But the first one's face is already sullen. She who counts, and measures, and calculates, and weighs. She who really is tired, but doesn't let go.

And the food comes to the table. Savory and inviting. She's anxious, trying to make quick calculations which will make it easier for her to eat. Quickly counting how much she ate today and promising herself that she won't eat till tomorrow. Only to get a quick approval, to eat while enjoying some inner peace before her self-doubt begins to work overtime. Before she begins suffering the wrath of the judgmental emotions swirling inside her, she closes her eyes for a moment, whispering promises, all sorts of promises. And drowns in eating. She'll savor it today. She'll be good tomorrow.

HOW DOES THE DIET LANGUAGE WORK?

It seems to us that we were always fluent in the Diet Language. We don't really distinguish ourselves from our authentic selves and the social and cultural marking that has affected the way this language came to be. We also don't really stop to ask ourselves what the nature of this language is and if speaking it does us good. We simply speak it, think it, feel it, act it. I assume that if this language led us to the coveted ideal of thinness we wouldn't even stop to discuss it, but recurring failure in achieving it and the tight bond linking happiness, health, and body weight creates a dissonance that causes us to grasp onto the Diet Language. A grasp that is almost indestructible. A grasp that is mainly attempts at control.

All of us humans use language. We describe, catalog, attribute, evaluate, talk, think, hear, read, write, dream, plan. People use it in the marketplace, on the street, in business meetings, in decisions of policy, between children and their parents, between neighbors, between friends, between lovers, between haters. Language has great importance in life. We speak differently to different people, we try to choose the right words and we sometimes get it wrong. It allows us to communicate with those far from us, to predict and establish the future, to solve complex problems, to develop laws that monitor our behavior and the behavior of others, to learn from other people or from cultures that no longer exist. It expresses ideas, meaning, messages or pieces of information that have developed and are stored within the psyche. It's a system of symbols which enables communicating ideas to another person's awareness, but it's also an autonomous system which creates a rich internal dialog.

The use of language is in two dimensions, external and internal. Through speaking, writing, dancing, singing, but also with thoughts, imagination, daydreams, planning, analyses, anxieties and fantasies. This language is unlike anything familiar. And it fills the mind with endless connections and verbal contexts. This is also how it creates suffering and maintains it as an inseparable part of life.

Every step along the life cycle brings us nearer to the end and creates suffering. A large part of this suffering is connected to things that are out of our control. We are born whether we want to or not. We grow old and frail and eventually die, like it or not. The finality of life creates suffering. But the sources of human suffering are not only based in those facts that are not under our control. The human mind, and the way it perceives the world, is the source of a considerable amount of the suffering we experience.

I invite you to peek into my own mind for a moment. Compared to the billions of people around the world, my life is perfectly fine. I have a family to love. A house to live in. Food to eat. A fascinating job which provides well and allows me to develop. Even so, not a day goes by when I don't experience at least one thought that causes me suffering, fear, and anxiety.

"Oh no, my throat is a bit sore, am I about to be sick?"

"I hope I won't be late for my meeting."

"Ugh, I have so many wrinkles."

"Are my kids okay? They haven't called all day."

"What if I don't get invited to the party?"

"He didn't answer my call. He's probably not interested in me."

"I'm so annoyed, I ate too much today. Now I'll definitely be fat."

"I'm worried that my son won't pass his test."

"They're probably talking about me. I feel excluded again."

This type of suffering can manifest itself in many ways. We are often afraid of what's to come, feel angry or sad, feel guilty, regret things that happened, get annoyed about physical pain, get anxious about changing plans, get bored, get nervous because of a traffic jam…and on and on.

Imagine yourselves going on a vacation with your significant other to a magical place. Greenery, ocean and blue skies, delicious food and tranquility. Everything seems to be good. But then trouble begins. Your mind starts to work. And you worry that maybe it's too good, and when will it end? What punishment will you get for it? What hard work awaits you when you return and you get annoyed about the humidity, and you actually miss a bit of a chill. And then, with everything objectively wonderful, you start worrying about the kids who stayed home alone, are filled with guilt that they stayed with the nanny while you're lying on the beach and indulging yourself. Immediately a thought hits you: maybe you're negligent parents? And suddenly you're overcome with longing for your kids and guilt that you're not with them, and you find yourselves packing up and rushing to leave.

That is the mind. It creates arbitrary contexts. Any stimulus, any object, any situation, any activity can be linked to any kind of negative emotion. Anywhere and anytime we can feel sadness and regret for what has long disappeared, fear what is not in front of us, worry about hypothetical dangers which it is doubtful if they will ever occur, compare everything to the alternative we fear or some coveted ideal. The mind tells stories, creates beliefs, myths, truths and values which it attaches to certain objects. And above all it mainly talks non-stop. It endlessly revolves like a giant carousel. One moment we feel smart, beautiful, talented, popular and successful and the next we're "shattered", ugly, rejected- a failure.

This consciousness is where pain is produced, because it cannot be locked away or put aside when we don't feel like listening to it or using it. It is always in action. Its nature is to yearn. A yearning that perpetuates the chase after pleasure and the escape from pain. A yearning that creates the experience of "not having", of absence, that causes suffering and keeps us forever preoccupied with what we don't have, what we could have, or what we deserve. We live with a constant sense of absence and an eternal feeling of "not having." This is also the sensation at the core of chasing after thinness and the escape from any weight which doesn't apply.

> *The Diet Language, like any other language, is duly run by our mind. It continues to do what it knows- talk non-stop, analyze, judge, compare, criticize, fantasize, tell stories, believe them, and manage itself according to them*

Let's take a look at Michal, one of my patients. She is 23 years old, and an education student. She told me this: "On Independence Day I was invited to a party, I got dressed, did my makeup, went to the party and I felt great. I danced, I drank, I felt popular. An hour went by and suddenly my ex-boyfriend, who I had broken up with two years earlier, arrived. I felt my heart suddenly pound with certain joy mixed with excitement, but at that same moment I realized that two years ago I weighed 4 kilos less. That wonderful sensation was immediately replaced with a sense of futility and failure. My whole night was ruined and I just wanted to disappear. I didn't want him to see me. To see how horrible I look."

Michal ruined for herself a wonderful night of dancing at a party just because she automatically latched on to the thought "Two years ago I weighed 4 kilos less." Grasping on to that thought led her to other thoughts. "Now my boyfriend is going to see how much weight I gained." "Now he's going to find out how bad I look." "I'm such a loser." "I'm worthless." "I look horrible." These thoughts ultimately told her "You have to run so he doesn't see you." This little story had a sad ending: Michal took her things, mumbled a lame excuse about a terrible headache, and left the party.

THE INTENSIVENESS OF THE MIND

I invite you to close your eyes. Just for a moment try to listen to your inner voice. Notice how the mind talks non-stop. It always has something to say, a comment, a question, about anything. Stop for a moment and try to think about your car for instance. What does your mind have to say about it? Now try to think about your parents for a moment. What does it have to say about them? The mind is at work. All the time. You don't have to do a thing. "I agree with that." "I like that." "That's true." "That's not true." "I don't know." "Really?" "I'm not sure I agree with him." It speaks and we listen. And believe every word.

What about the body? And eating? The mind, which speaks the Diet Language, takes visual representations that stem from culture, society, history, education, and the relationship between them and makes everything that is negative or linked to negativity accessible and available. In this way, almost anything can trigger suffering. The weight that hasn't changed, eating a pizza that wasn't on the designated menu, a struggle to be thin, or gaining weight after a diet, a boyfriend that we think has left only because we gained weight.

The Diet Language causes a lot of suffering

JUST LET ME NOT GET HUNGRY AND WANT TO EAT

He had post gastric sleeve surgery and already has dropped 25 kilos. Anxiety consumes him. "Just let me not get hungry." "Just let me lose enough weight." "Just let me not experience failure." "Just let the hunger hormone stay away and not undermine my control." "Just keep the joy of eating from returning." And so the days go by and he "celebrates" every day

70

when he manages to eat so little. Every day when the food didn't taste good.

He is 30 years old and already has fifteen years of dieting behind him. He has a little boy, a sweet wife, an interesting job... and yet he's busy despising his body. Or actually, himself. And anxiety fools him. For a moment it promises him success if he avoids food. And for a moment it's angry that he didn't listen to his body's signals. And he's in the middle, trapped. Confused. Wondering, "Am I allowed to eat or not?" He's a man of science, preoccupied with the caloric balance. Input and output. "That's the way to do it," he said. That's what he was taught and that's what he does. Sticking to the Diet Language. Before it made him binge, feel guilty and angry, but now it wore a different guise. Complete abstinence. This way and the other are the same. They only ensure that what he fears most-weight gain-happens.

The thought machine continues to do what it does best: babble. He's lost amidst his thoughts as they talk non-stop. Blaming, planning, comparing, being angry. He's used to this mind consuming suffering and he has trouble giving it up.

Just let me not be hungry, just let me not want to eat. Every day that goes by without him eating is almost directly accounted as a good day in his book. Eating a cookie, on the other hand, ruins everything and makes it a bad day. And pleasure from eating? That's a dirty word. Enjoying himself is not allowed. He has to suffer or he'll gain weight. "Just let me not be hungry." He's always alert to his body's signals. Dreading the sensations of hunger and craving. It's hard for him to understand that trying to escape food and the joy of it is what is making him gain weight.

Today he ate a slice of bread with hummus. Just like that, a slice of bread with hummus. He ate it slowly. Mindfully, attentively. Fully allowing the pleasure, the fullness and the satiation following it. And as strange as it may seem, he was a bit relieved. And he even dared to say it tasted good.

And the thoughts were there as usual. Criticizing, judging, cautioning, warning... and he, so used to them, is having trouble letting go.

THE WAY THE DIET LANGUAGE CREATES SUFFERING

"When you delude yourself that you see something, you presume that everyone else see it. But reality is not external. It exists in the human mind, and nowhere else." [39]

Many are convinced that food must be feared, that you have to exercise a lot to lose weight, that you have to count calories, and routinely weigh yourself. Many people are mistaken, confusing how they think about reality and its true nature. This confusion creates suffering.

The Diet Language is so inherent to our lives that it is hard to look at objectively. Here I will try to expose it for what it really is and show you how it has confused the areas most intuitive to us as human beings; and how it has taken away our freedom and inner authority.

In order to do so we will begin with a short exercise: Sit comfortably, lean back in your chair, and relax your arms and legs. Place your feet on the floor by your chair and try to close your eyes. Follow the rhythm of your breaths. The air going in and out. Note the sounds entering the room. Look inside yourselves and try to listen to what your thoughts are telling you, what emotions are wandering in and what sensations your body is signaling. Note the clothes you chose to wear today. Note the way in which your body is arranged in the chair, the way you feel about it. What part of it do you feel? What does this sensation make you feel? Do you like your body? Have you ever dieted? What age did you start? What did you weigh when you went on your first diet? What do you weigh today? How many diets did you go on along the way? Do you count calories? How long have you been weighing yourself? What do you feel as I ask you these questions?

Do you like standing in front of the mirror? What do you say to yourself as you stand before it? What does it say to you? How many times do you want to eat something and you withhold yourself from eating it? How much time do you spend during the day thinking about what you've eaten, how much, and what you're going to eat? How significant a role do these questions play in your thoughts? To what extent do they run your life? Where did this lead you to? To what extent does it make you feel good about the food you eat, your body, and the clothes you wear?

Stay with those thoughts running through your head and slowly return to the present. When you're ready to, you may open your eyes. Stay with your thoughts for a few minutes more, then write them down.

Next to each thought you wrote down, try to write-what behavior does it trigger for you? What does it make you do, feel? Did these behaviors lead you to feel better about your body? About eating? About yourselves? Did these feelings persist in the short-term? In the long run?

Now try to say what you wrote down out loud. What do you feel now?

Ask yourselves again:

- Are these thoughts familiar?
- How do these thoughts affect eating behavior?
- Are these thoughts helpful?
- How do you benefit from holding on to these thoughts?
- How much suffering did you experience when these thoughts came to you? How much vitality?
- To what extent were these behaviors effective in the short-term? In the long run?
- Do these thoughts help you become who you want to be?

ATTEMPTS TO CONTROL WEIGHT AND EATING ARE THE PROBLEM AND NOT THE SOLUTION

Control is a command, a restriction, a law meant to manage behavior or actions. Control requires investing time, energy, resources, and directing certain actions toward deliberate results. This strategy does indeed work in many life situations. For instance, most people try to avoid situations that may end in accidents, injury, or death. Most of them run when these things occur. If we see a dangerous animal, an erupting volcano, or a river overflowing, we run.

These controlling behaviors are corresponding, and on many occasions effective, and there is nothing dysfunctional about them. Even attempts to control behavior that is intended to prevent or minimize physical pain is accepted and found to be effective in many cases. For instance, we'll take a painkiller for a headache. We'll go to the doctor if we have a sore throat, we'll rest to feel more energized, we'll exercise to feel better. But did these attempts at control prove themselves when it comes to the mind's illusions? For instance, if we have a panic attack which manifests itself in a cold sweat, stress, an increased heart rate and an intense need to pace back and forth, we'll tend to develop techniques that supposedly protect us from experiencing anxiety. If it seems to us that a certain place, experience, or person triggered the attack, we'll do anything to avoid any situation that may remind us of that same event, person, or sensation. We will start living with an intense need to avoid anything that we think may lead to an anxiety attack. Life will become a system of avoidances that allegedly protects us from one experience but creates actual suffering for us in countless other areas of life. We'll avoid going abroad, going to crowded places, being alone, or other things.

What we invented as the solution for a problem sometimes becomes the problem itself. In many senses this is the fate we meet with diets, which we have created to help us flee from the fear of gaining weight. Attempting to control what cannot be controlled regarding our bodies has become harmful, damaging, and fattening.

The list of control strategies is massive. I will mention but a few: avoiding certain foods, self-punishment, exercise, avoiding going to the beach, not eating after a certain hour, avoiding going out to restaurants, prohibiting foods that are deemed fattening, or avoiding buying clothes. Behind every strategy is a belief that maintains it. "A diet creates a structure that will help me control food better and lose weight." "I will be able to develop a real relationship only if I lose weight." "There are good foods and bad foods." "Food affects how I look and my attractiveness." "Punishments encourage me to watch my weight." "I'm not worthy of recognition in social events because of my heavy weight." "You have to eat breakfast." "Only one piece of candy is allowed a day." "You should never eat between meals." "You have to put one teaspoon of oil in your salad." "No dessert." "You have to eat a lot of vegetables." "Pizza is allowed only once a week." "Don't eat at night." "You have to lose weight and be thin." Every person has a list of rules and beliefs that they have created for themselves.

> *The diet is a control strategy that we have invented as the solution for obesity which, with time, has become the problem*

Weight is also a control strategy. It has become a vital tool for supervising the body. It has become the authority which evaluates and measures the person and his behavior. Its role is not limited to mirroring the situation, since it always acts as the critic or the judge. Because of this role, it does not only examine and evaluate past behavior, but also manages and affects our behavior in the future. The use of it has created countless rituals, behaviors, beliefs, and thoughts that are solely meant to control. Many of my patients would get on the scale and suck in their stomach, not eat before being weighed, take off all their clothes, or make sure to always get weighed on the same day and hour. Some came up with secret prayers, come in the same outfit they dubbed "weigh in clothes," and more. For speakers of the Diet Language weight is the tyrant. It manages our eating, our feelings, and mainly rates our value in our own eyes and in the eyes of others. But it has also become a double edged sword. We fear it, run away from it, cheat it. It is sometimes found to be an effective dictator in the short-term, but in the long run it usually fails.

Weight is a control strategy which is sometimes effective in the short-term; in the long run it is harmful and fattening.

What's important for continuing our discussion is recognizing the fact that for most people, eating governed by control and the wish to lose weight will always be restrictive and dietetic, which is destined to end in physical torment and regaining lost weight. In reality, 95% of people trying to lose weight gain it back within one to five years from completing their weight loss program.

The problem with diets extends beyond mere failure to achieve weight loss, however:

- Diets are fattening- 95% of people who lose weight regain it within five years, sometimes with additional weight.
- Healthy eating has become a synonym for dietetic and slimming and has lost its value as an essential tool for good health.
- The dialog with food has gone away and it is now conducted out of fear, dichotomy, stipulation,

prohibition, abstinence, threat, and mysticism.

- Attention to hunger and satiation has been lost.
- An irreversible blow to body image and self-esteem has been inflicted. This type of harm exposes the person to abuse, using addictive substances, mental disorders, and eating disorders.
- Harmful processes are taking place on a social and health level, stemming from the medicalization and mystification of weight gain and eating. For example:
  o A sharp increase in social discrimination based on body shape and weight.
  o Unhealthy food being sold in the guise of being healthy and dietetic.
- Living life according to a list of things to avoid.
- Amplifying obesity.
- Weight control techniques simply don't work. They may bring momentary relief, but in the long run they only lead to renewed weight gain.

The Diet Language is a language which causes much suffering. It makes us live an entire life outside of life.

CLINGING TO THE DIET LANGUAGE

The Diet Language, as we have seen, is a language with its own words, its own sentences, and its own dialog. It is perceived by many as an absolute truth that we must behave in accordance with.

Here is an exercise to demonstrate how stuck we are on the Diet Language: take the palms of your hands, which in this exercise represent your thoughts, and look at the world through them. Cover your eyes with them and please ask yourself the following questions:

- What does the world look like?
- What's it like to walk around all day with your hands covering your eyes?
- How much does this limit you?
- How does this restrict your ability to respond to the world?
- Or your ability to communicate with the world?

Now let's try this in the world of diets, food, and weight. Imagine your hands covering your eyes, and they are full of opinions, stories, thoughts, and feelings, all of them speaking from the Diet Language:

- "Look at yourself"
- "Can't you get your act together and lose some weight?"
- "You're such a loser"
- "No guy's ever going to want you"
- "Why did you need that cake?"

Through the screen of the Diet Language the world is seen in calories and kilograms. Sticking to this kind of thought makes the us see this as:

- The one and only truth
- Instructions or orders that must be followed or obeyed
- A horror that he or she must get rid of as soon as possible
- Something important that requires all of your attention
- Something that you cannot let go of even if it ruins your life
- Something that is happening, right now, even if it seems to be related to the past or future

This is exactly how the Diet Language runs our lives. It is embedded within us and we live by it.

We're afraid to let it go and we justify it in a reasonable and convincing manner. We think that if we let go of this language we'll lose weight. We can't see that absurdly enough, despite years of clinging on to it, we have actually gained weight. We tend to say that if everyone is doing it we must be doing something wrong. This tightens our grip on the Diet Language. And our inner critic explains to us very convincingly that we just lack will power and motivation and we should try a bit harder. The mind, as we have seen, does an excellent job. It whips out explanations that sound convincing, and explains with the utmost logic why we simply have to keep holding on tight to the Diet Language.

The automatic clinging to the Diet Language also gives rise to heavy guilt. Guilt that is an unrealistic expectation that we could have and should have acted differently. "Why didn't I restrain myself?" "Why do I have no character?" "Why did we buy that good bread for the house?"…we have a hard time giving up this guilt. It seems to us that it watches us so we'll be better, more perfect. That if we don't punish ourselves, we'll receive an even greater punishment. Guilt is an excellent way to show us how fear takes control, and governs us.

We grasp on to thoughts telling us: "As long as I'm fat I'll never deserve to be treated well." "I'm worthless." "As long as I'm fat, I'll never have a significant other." "Fat is unhealthy." Our lives become narrow and packed with endless negative thoughts like, "what did I eat, how much, and how do I lose weight?" Like a geometric series the thoughts run through the mind. One thought births the next and they get more and more entangled in one another. They become a spider web which traps us. These thoughts lead to various behaviors. For example:

A

- Pizza is a fattening and dangerous food
- I'm not allowed to eat pizza
- I must avoid pizza
- I want to eat pizza so bad
- Everybody's having it, I want some too (Dissonance- fear vs. desire. The wish to eat vs. the fear to eat)
- Yay, I managed to avoid eating/ Yay, that pizza was amazing
- Oh, what a disappointment
- I have to give up
- But maybe I will have some, it's so tempting and delicious
- No, I can't, I know
- I can't resist
- Okay, I'll have some, just today
- I'll eat a lot, I have to go back on my diet tomorrow anyway
- Bingeing
- Gaining weight

B

- Fat children have no will power and they are not intelligent
- If I have a fat child it means I'm not a good parent
- I have to try to help my child to lose weight
- If he doesn't lose weight he'll suffer like me
- If he doesn't lose weight he won't have any friends
- Obesity is dangerous
- The child isn't succeeding in losing weight
- What does this say about me

- I'm such an unsuccessful parent
- What an unsuccessful child
- I'm just a bad parent
- I'm quite ashamed of my child
- The child is ashamed of himself
- The child closes himself off
- Loses his confidence
- Eats more
- Gains weight

C

- No man wants a fat woman
- No man will want me
- I have to lose weight
- I'm just a loser, I can't do it
- "Nobody wants me"
- Why should I try, I can't do it
- I shouldn't bother buying clothes
- I shouldn't bother dating
- I'm just worthless
- Sadness and depression
- Loneliness
- Binge eating
- Weight gain

When we cling on to the Diet Language, we sink deep into a "word grinder". Our eating becomes defective, our self-esteem is low and we often find ourselves in an almost constant process of weight gain. Our world becomes governed by cognitive rumination- "intellectual regurgitation." We find ourselves trying to understand, to evaluate, to find reasons or to examine possible outcomes of our behavior. And thus we slowly ground to nothing.

> *The Diet Language grinds us down to nothing. It doesn't cease lecturing us, following us, judging us, governing us*

COGNITIVE ENTANGLEMENT IN THE DIET LANGUAGE

A person who has dieted and lost weight will constantly be preoccupied with thoughts telling him, "I'm not allowed to eat ice cream." "This time I have to maintain my achievement." "This time I'm going to succeed." "I have to exercise regularly." "How many calories did I eat today?" "Oh no, I gained an entire kilo. I have to lose it by tomorrow." "Today I'll only eat a tiny bit." The deeper he delves into this thinking, the more intensive his preoccupation with eating will become. He will experience this as an essential way to watch his weight, which will usually be detrimental to him, because this intensified preoccupation will lead him to binges, causing him to gain weight. After he's gained it, he'll become entangled in a new set of thoughts: "I'm so weak-willed." "How did I let this happen this time?" "I promised myself that this time I'll keep it off forever." "I have to start again and lose the weight." "What diet will I try now?" "How will I keep it off this time?" and again, endless preoccupation and entanglement with weight, food, eating, and body, which creates great suffering.

In professional circles, this thought mill is called cognitive entanglement. This entanglement, by retouching the same subjects that preoccupy us about food, diet, and weight, over and over again, intensifies the problem. It causes a negative mood, a constant reentering into the diet cycles (yo-yo cycles), direct suffering because of the adherence to thoughts and because of the behavior this adherence creates and accelerates.

THE DIET LANGUAGE AND THE EXPERIENTIAL AVOIDANCE

Our day to day reality is tinted by thoughts, beliefs, and stories we tell ourselves. Among the speakers of the Diet Language, reality is tinted by a lot of pain, anxiety, guilt and fear. In order to handle these emotions, we adopt creative ways of changing them, their frequency and the reasons we believe lead to them. We try in every possible way to escape them and to avoid experiencing them or anything we see as related to them or triggering them. Those attempts at escape that seem to us like a fitting method of coping are what we call experiential avoidance. They are driven by a fear to experience the same threatening psychological events which are impossible to contain.

At times these avoidances are efficient and effective, but many times they may create endless problems of their own.

I'll describe it this way: if there's a wolf behind the door we can throw stones at it, shoot it, or hide. If it's snowing we can wear a coat, or stay somewhere warm and dry. But what is true for events that occur outside does not necessarily apply to events that take place within the mind. There are many ways to escape, which we use intentionally or unintentionally when scary thoughts, emotions and situations which we have a hard time dealing with, appear:

- We worry
- We rehash the past
- We fantasize about the future
- We imagine escape scenarios
- We imagine revenge scenarios
- We imagine suicidal scenarios
- We think about how unfair this is

- We think about "if only…"
- We blame ourselves
- We blame others
- We blame the world
- We reason with ourselves
- We speak positively to ourselves
- We speak negatively to ourselves
- We analyze ourselves (trying to understand why we are the way we are)
- We analyze the situation (why did it happen as it happened)
- We analyze others (why they are like they are)

In my clinic I meet many people who use food to solve problems or avoid feelings they find difficult to experience like boredom, loneliness, anger, and guilt. At first glance it seems that it is a great technique, but it turns out that it can cause intense pain and suffering. After all, once we eat we are left with the initial problem, and we only added to our inner torment by feeling guilty over using food to try to escape from what we are feeling. Reality proves to us that when we try to avoid difficult and scary feelings and experiences, our suffering can continue to grow.

The fear of experiencing excess weight also births various ways to escape it, like avoiding eating, employing calorie burning techniques, avoiding events where food is served, avoiding certain foods, intense physical activity, weight loss programs, reclusiveness, or otherwise limiting social contact, and more. These may seem effective at first, but in the long run, they only amplify the problem we fear. Our attempts to run from certain stimuli takes us near it and its possible consequences, making them more "real." Many people who are trapped in the cycle of diets and fear of weight gain are sunk deep in binge eating, loss of control over their eating habits, low self-esteem, recurring adherence to diets and weight gain.

> *Avoidance is usually effective in the short-term, but in the long run it becomes a double edged sword*

For instance, if we avoid going to a party mainly because we think we are fat and clumsy and unattractive and we're convinced that no outfit looks good on us, at first we will experience some relief because we escaped experiences and feelings that threaten us, but eventually this avoidance will enhance our feeling of incompatibility, and leave us sad and lonely..

The situation becomes more complicated, because every thought, memory, feeling, impulse or sensation, every object or situation which are not perceived as negative at their base can become the target of avoidance. A restaurant, shopping, going to the beach, a friend from a certain point in life, a family meal, a wedding, the sense of being alone, a happy sensation...We can find ourselves investing tremendous efforts in our attempt to control internal events which we perceive as negative. This preoccupation becomes a real "full-time job" (albeit a decidedly unpleasant and unrewarding one). We get in over our heads during our nearly constant attempts to ward off the problems that are bothering us, to the point we put our lives "on hold." We usually comfort ourselves by saying that when we "get over" our problems or "solve" them, we could finally live life again and fulfill our goals. "When I'll lose weight I'll find love." "I'm not going to the beach until I'm skinny."

Attempts to avoid weight-related feelings and emotions can be categorized into three main groups: avoiding the experience of excess weight, avoiding eating "bad" foods, and avoiding gaining weight.

Avoiding feeling excess weight- Avoidance of this manifests itself in many ways. The most common one is adhering to dieting despite knowing they're a failure out of a hidden belief that "Maybe I can be the one to prove the statistics wrong." This adherence causes us to persist and try nearly any possible way to achieve the dream. The result: entering the cycle of gaining and losing weight (the yo-yo cycle) and everything it implies.

Avoiding eating and avoiding gaining weight through it- In dieting, many foods are marked as forbidden. Eating itself is restricted, controlled, liable to rules and restrictions and accompanied by fear, guilt, and a sense of sin. It causes an almost constant need to avoid encountering "forbidden" foods. The battle against temptation and the accompanying guilt weigh heavily on us and we feel as if we're jailed behind internal and external bars-Those we force upon ourselves and those society forces upon us. And again the result of this avoidance is the same. The short-term profit is clear- we avoid scary foods, avoid feeling threatening emotions, and so on. But in the long-term, these bars can cause isolation, sadness, and even depression. This may increase the occurrence of emotional eating and bring on what we most wanted to escape: weight gain. These situations may nurture behaviors that will lead to more and more diets, causing loss of control, binge eating, and regaining weight. Binges are also a type of avoidance. They become nearly the only way to eat "forbidden" foods. A binge is supposedly the only way to eat without "seeing" you're eating.

> *Avoiding eating leads to loss of control and binges*

Avoiding life itself - Reclusiveness and avoiding social encounters, restaurants, shopping for clothes, the beach, doctors' appointments, looking at the mirror...all of these are situations which makes individuals avoid sensing their bodies and acknowledging them. In the long run, people in these situations become reclusive, angry, and depressed.

They are sitting on the fence, waiting, thinking: "When I'll be thin then…I'll get to know life, I'll buy clothes, I'll go abroad, I'll look for a new job, I'll go sailing. I'll live."

These attempts at escape and avoidance may lead to reclusiveness, deficient nutrition and disrupted eating, a strict lifestyle, wasting money on weight loss programs, loss of true life values, adhering to diets, a distorted eating dialog which mirrors other dialogs in life, depression, low self-esteem, and weight gain.

THE 13 YEAR OLD BOY

His hair flops over his face. The black sweatshirt hangs loose on his body. It is 32 degrees outside. He is 13 years old. He lives in a small town in the north of Israel.

He spends 200 of the 365 days of the year at home. Locked in his room, hunched over the computer. Day has become night and night is day. He doesn't make up excuses about not wanting to go to school anymore. He is now closed off in his room. There he sleeps, watches shows on the computer, and eats. McDonald's, sometimes hummus, and a lot of pizzas. That's the menu. And just dare to say no to him. His grades have dropped below 60 and his friends have given up on him and faded away. The door is closed. No one goes in or comes out.

His mother is losing her mind. She's convinced his weight is what is stopping him from living. And she's not exactly wrong. 95 kilos is a lot. And she counts for him, and tests him. Tries to cook for him. Pushes him on. Willing to do anything if he'll only lose weight. Deep down he knows there's nothing he can do. He can't be told what to do and be followed about and have his eating managed. Even if it is all done with good intentions. The feeling he is getting from this is that he is simply a failure. And he is only 13 years old.

THE DIET LANGUAGE AND AVOIDING LIVING IN THE HERE AND NOW

Living life according to the in the Diet Language makes it difficult to live in the here and now. It is a life which is largely experienced from a perspective that is tinted by calories, kilograms, chasing after an "ideal" weight, and a constant struggle with food. Thus it becomes a life that is almost constantly focused on the past or the future. People who are governed by the Diet Language are greatly preoccupied with memories of what was: What they weighed in the past, eating plans that led to weight loss. They miss how they weighed when they were 20, the dress that is waiting in the closet, or the lover they had then. At the same time they're busy contemplating and making plans for the future. They constantly fear what will happen if they don't lose weight or fantasize about what will happen when they do lose it. They often simply wait for a miracle that will redeem them from a few kilograms with a belief that this will change their lives. That they will be able to do all those things that they have avoided. By so doing, life only passes them by.

> *A life that is governed by the Diet Language is a life lived mostly with yearning for what was and fantasizing about what will be*

CLINGING TO THE DIET LANGUAGE HURTS VALUES

Our values- the way we want to behave, our idea about what kind of people we want to be, what type of powers and qualities we want to develop- these values are our compass. They are the stepping stones on the path we choose to take.

We sometimes mistake goals for values. Goals, big as they may be, provide concrete points we can navigate to, but the value is the way there. The process that is never achieved or finished. It is a common mistake to think that values, like goals, are in the future. Values regard the present.

Those of us who speak the Diet Language believe in the thin ideal. Low body weight becomes a value which pushes aside other values. We adopt it not out of free will. It is forced upon us and governs our lives. It leads us to dieting, avoiding certain foods, wasting a lot of money, disrupted eating, self-negligence, self-hatred , damaging relationships, and depression. Along the way our other values are harmed, including freedom, development, good relationships, self-love, intimacy, taking care of ourselves, health, inner freedom, free choice, friendship and joy.

THE DIET LANGUAGE AND SELF-LABELING

The story we tell ourselves about who we are and what we are is a complex story. It has objective facts like age and sex, family situation, profession, and it also has description, judging, and evaluating the game of life, relationships, strong and weak points, hopes, and dreams. If we speak the Diet Language, the story we tell ourselves is full of details about how many kilograms we weigh, and the sizes of our waists, breasts, buttocks, and thighs. We link our identity to our status regarding weight. A strict adherence to defining ourselves through the Diet Language keeps us from daring to define the true life values by which we'd want to live and prevents us from moving towards them.

> *The Diet Language measures a person's value in kilograms. We believe happiness has a value, too, however*

DIETING AGAIN

She shed crocodile tears. "I'll never give up," she claimed. Even when each time she succeeds, she only keeps her weight off for only two months before it starts up again, going a bit higher each time. And now she's already at eighty kilos...but, "I'll never give up." And she has good reason to. In front of the mirror, in front of the closet, in front of boys...that belly that even when she's lying down is big and thick and full of wrinkles. "How can I live like this?" she said. It's true that she never weighed eighty kilos, and she can see that since her first diet at the age of 12 she's slowly diminishing, moving between a few moments of happiness and many moments of despair...but it's all or nothing for her...so maybe she should gain weight only in order to ultimately have a weight reduction operation?

"A diet again?" I asked "Again you'll lose 20 kilos, be thin for two months, and gain it back? That's the story of your life," I added. "Right" she said, "but I can't give up. I just can't."

She is 22 years old. She has wonderful parents who shower her with their love and care. She also has good friends.In fact, everything seems good. Except for the weight. If only she was thin... if only she had a boyfriend. If only, if only...

Her life goes on, and she's suffering. Not letting go. And her beautiful smile is twisted into wrinkled angles, and the glow of youth fades. and yet she still does not let go.

THE DIET LANGUAGE CREATES STIGMAS, PREJUDICE AND WEIGHT DISCRIMINATION

A story is told about an old Chinese woman who had two large urns. Each urn was hung on the end of a stick she balanced on her neck. One of the urns was cracked and while the other urn, which was perfect, always carried the full amount of water on the long way from the river to the house, the cracked urn always arrived only half full. Thus the old woman only brought home only one and a half urns of water. The perfect urn was proud of its achievements while the cracked urn was poor and miserable. It was ashamed of its imperfection and of the fact that it was only able to do half of the work it was meant to do. One day at the river, after two years of feeling like a complete failure, the cracked urn turned to the old woman and said to her, "I'm ashamed of myself; because of my cracks the water drips all the way from the river to your house." The old woman smiled and replied: "Have you noticed there are flowers along the way?" (folk tale)

"Last night a lot of children were seen on the screen. And children, as you know, always steal the show. But these specific ones probably stole the McDonald's milkshake machine. There were carbohydrate shocked teenagers who made baggy pants look like skinny jeans. Girls that once they parted from the stroller turned into one. Seven year old boys who whose bodies clearly show...that they need an appointment with someone from the Kmart undergarment department to fit them with a bra.." (Yedioth Achronot- "Weight of the Nation", Assaf Weiss, 29.11.12)

"A woman in her thirties who was admitted at the "Shiba" Medical Center at Tel-Hashomer in labor claims she experienced unprecedented humiliation from the anesthesiologist who treated her. He said: "disgusting fatty, do something about yourself," the new mother accused on the hospital's Facebook page. "I was humiliated on the most exciting day of my life." The hospital's response: "If anything irregular happened, we will take disciplinary action." (Channel 2 news, 29.4.2012)

"Shachaf Kishnia will never forget this humiliation. Shachaf, a 22 year old young lady from Bat-Yam, arrived at Wolfson Hospital in Holon this January in an attempt to discover the source of the intense abdominal pain she had been suffering from for some time. She never imagined that there of all places, in the Surgical A Department of the veteran governmental hospital, she would be ridiculed by her caregivers, that her examination would force her to lie on the examination table for a long while and listen as the medical staff mocked her weight. A stunned Shachaf had nothing to do but close her eyes and try to stop the tears. During the entire examination, the head of the department and the medical team stood around her bed like a band of fools, laughing and making disparaging, humiliating and insulting comments, claims Shachaf in a law suit she has filed against the Department of Health." (Article by Ran Reznik, Israel Hayom, October, 2012)

These stories are just a small selection which illustrate the scornful attitudes society now displays towards weight.

In the field of public health, stigma is a familiar enemy. All through history there have been many cases in which suffering was forced on groups that were suspect to certain diseases in order to "encourage" treatment and prevention. In this context, the stigma is an implication which says:"You are responsible for your disease. You are immoral, unclean, and lazy, that's why you contracted it." This was how Africans were blamed for tuberculosis, homosexuals for AIDS, and women for hysteria.

The stigma attached to people with obesity reaches people of all ages, races, and sexes and follows them from the day they are born untill the day they die. In the Diet Language, the stigma attached to people with obesity links various traits with excess weight: laziness, lack of intelligence, weakness, lack of willpower, and failure. These stereotypes are deeply rooted and lead to discrimination which invades every possible field. It is expressed in teasing, using hurtful names, inflicting physical harm, or preventing equal treatment in hiring for work, being promoted at work, providing services, in medical care, at schools, how the media treats people with obesity,and in how parents educate their children about their body weight.. According to recent estimations, the rate of weight discrimination in the U.S alone has gone up by 66% in the last decade[40] and can now be compared to rates of racial discrimination (although there are no recent studies about this problem in Israel since it has not yet been brought to the public's awareness, but the findings would likely be similar).

> *The stigma stems from the mistaken perception that our weight is under our full control and responsibility. According to this perception, we are to blame for our excess weight!*

What intensifies weight discrimination is the policy of the War on Obesity. A policy that has embraced the principals of the War on Smoking and attempts to implement them when dealing with obesity. A policy that believes that regulation and intimidation will cause changes in behavior that will lead to people sticking to a healthy lifestyle. A lifestyle that will lead to normal body weight by BMI standards.

A policy that is convinced that controlling eating is possible and fitting and will bring to weight loss and health. This is a policy that speaks the Diet Language and defines any fat person as ill or potentially ill, as responsible for his disease, and as someone who must be acted for and against until he loses weight.

THE STIGMA AMONG CHILDREN AND YOUTH

In a society in which thinness is a value attributed to success, happiness and health, obesity will always be a testament of failure, lack of sympathy, and illness. The stigma connected to body weight begins at an early age. There is evidence now of discriminatory treatment of kids as young as three.

A number of studies have examined the stigma against overweight school children from kindergarten through elementary school. They showed that children, like adults, regard an overweight child as having the ability to control his or her situation, and the more control over the situation is attributed to him, the more negative the stereotypes and prejudice against him become. A survey held in 2012 among first grade students in 29 Oklahoma schools demonstrated that a child with overweight is the most disliked among his peers.

In a different study[41] held in 2004 among 42 kindergarteners aged four to six, it was found that the child with overweight had the most negative character traits attributed to him: mean, stupid, and ugly. He was also attributed negative behaviors: lacking friends, being messy looking, and being obnoxious. These beliefs led to social rejection of the child with overweight. When the children were asked to choose who they would most want as a friend from a series of pictures of children with thin/normal weight/overweight, 55% chose the thin child, 38% chose the child with normal weight and only 7% chose the child with overweight.

Among teenagers the situation is similar. A study[42] published in 2011 showed that among 41% of teens, excess weight is the number one cause for bullying, ridicule, and humiliation, and as body weight increases, the child becomes more vulnerable.

There are countless ways in which teens hurt children with overweight. They ridicule them, call them names, make vicious comments, tease them during physical activity, ignore them, bully them, exclude them from activities, spread negative rumors about them, threaten them, and physically harm them.

The problem becomes even more severe when the discrimination invades the home- the one place that is supposed to protect the child or teenager most of all. Within the home, discrimination usually disguises itself. The parents belittle one another, the mother stipulates different requests with weight loss ("You can get a guitar if you lose five kilos"), parents and siblings constantly observing how the child eats- what's on the plate, what he ate, what he took out of the fridge. This all ammounts to a regime of constant criticism and judgment. Many parents feel that the weight of their child is a testimony of how good of a parent they are. A child with overweight means they are failure as parents. If the parents themselves are with overweight, they try to protect their child from suffering it.. Some parents are preoccupied with how they look through how their children look. Many mistakenly think that by criticizing and badgering on one front and dieting and lifestyle change on the other they will succeed in getting the child's weight to change. And in order to achieve this goal it seems as if every option is viable. Forced physical activity, weight loss groups, restrictions and punishments, invading their plate by overt and covert methods, and making comments like "Didn't you have enough? Look at yourself!" "You're allowed one piece of candy a day." "I don't allow pizza." These comments are often said in a threatening and strict manner and they negate the child's inner freedom and his attention to his body. They undermine his ability to get to know himself and his needs and trust his abilities. This surveillance of the child's eating habits is manifested in a stern expression, scary, piercing eyes, and constant disapproval. Many children experience this kind of emotional abuse on a daily basis.

A study published in 2013 examined 918 parents of children aged 2-18. The findings showed that excess weight was the main reason for nagging the child, regardless of the weight of the parents or the child[43].

Here are some of the things told to me by kids in the clinic:

- "Mommy doesn't hug me. When she comes to take me from kindergarten the first thing she asks me is what I ate and why did I eat so much."

- "I most like to eat alone in my room with no one there to count or measure."

- "I know my mother is always spying on me. I always feel guilty. I hate myself because I know I steal food."

- "I wasn't picked for soccer again. I choked down my tears and said I didn't even want to play."

- "My mother pulled me from kindergarten because I'd come home crying every day. The kids laughed at me in class, on the playground, even on the way home. When I came home I was in hysterics."

- "My mother says to me, 'You eat so much, look at yourself, nothing fits you'. She doesn't understand how much she hurts me. As if I eat to spite her. Doesn't she understand that this is how I am?"

Statistics published by the Rudd Institute at the University of Connecticut show that in parents' perception, 53% of bullied and harassed children are linked to excess weight. This report is in line with a survey held among teens showing that in their eyes, 40% of bullying is the result of excess weight. The population of children with overweight and obesity are a specifically weakened group. The child, experiencing pain inflicted upon him by his peers and his family members finds himself entrapped. A study[44] examining 4,746 children with overweight found that 47% of girls with obesity and 34% of boys with obesity suffer from teasing about weight from their family members. Even in cases in which the parent does not directly discriminate against his own child, but belittles children or other people with overweight, the child still thinks it is directed at him.

This discrimination intensifies as a result of exposure to media- cinema, video games, television, social networks and fashion magazines. The news media has great power in shaping the audience's minds. The study shows that seeing images has a greater effect on shaping perception than reading or hearing.

Statistics published by the Rudd[45] Institute at the University of Connecticut in 2011 show that the media "specializes" in portraying the person with overweight in a negative to derogatory manner. And what's true for adults is true for children and adolescents as well. Today they are exposed to unilateral media, sending out messages creating an atmosphere of de-legitimization of a variety of different weights and body shapes. In recent decades there have been more thin and less overweight characters in animated films.

An extensive discussion has developed over the last year about this issue following the process of slimming down Minnie Mouse that has occurred in Walt Disney movies over the years. In many movies, thin characters are depicted as the more attractive ones. They take action for the common good, they're more intelligent, they're young, happy, loving, and good. Overweight characters are depicted as less attractive. Today no one wants to be identified with obesity. And children constantly exposed to content that favors thinness in the media take on these preferences. From an early age they grow up with the feeling that they're illegitimate. That they are unworthy. They go out into the world with this feeling. And the world treats them accordingly.

Children are the most vulnerable part of the world's population. They are affected from both inside and outside the home. The wish to change them so they fit in with the thin ideal disrupts their growth process and permanently damages self-esteem. This is how the right to grow into their bodies and into a healthy, confident adult, is robbed from them

---

A SECOND RATE CHILD

The most painful kind of discrimination is the one a parent inflicts upon their child. It is a kind of covert discrimination. A confusing one. The parent only wants the good of the child. And he tells him "What, you think I want to harm you? I just want you to be happy. Maybe you'll make a little effort not to eat that chocolate bar? I don't understand how many schnitzels you need, you eat more than I do, no wonder you're fat." All the while, the child has his head down, feeling ashamed, guilty. He's convinced his parents are right and he's just not trying hard enough. He swears that come tomorrow he'll take better care to keep his parents happy with him. But he can't do it, again. Food tempts him, calls him, promises all kinds of promises of pleasure and experience and he can't help himself, and all the promises he made to himself quickly disappear. Then he begins stealing again, feeling guilty again... and disappointing his parents again.

Sometimes the parents that want good for their

child will take him for a "walk" or hire a personal trainer for him and add, "We work so hard for you and you make no effort." They will find it hard to understand that their child may not like physical activity; maybe he prefers playing chess or the piano. And he is pained by his failure. His struggle against his body is so difficult for him. He really is trying hard, at least he feels that he is. The child has no one to talk to, for who can relate to him? His parents who insist that he must lose weight for his own good are not approachable.He sinks deeper into himself. Doesn't talk a lot, doesn't eat with everyone, preferring toeat in hiding instead. He has to watch himself, not eat too much candy...he hides away, wears large t-shirts. Doesn't take his shirt off at the beach, doesn't see his friends. And his parents, who were supposed to support him, to love and protect him, are pushing him away.

STIGMA AND DISCRIMINATION IN THE ADULT POPULATION

With age, weight discrimination increases. A survey[46] of 2,449 women with overweight and obesity points to the fact that the people who cause weight discrimination are surprisingly those who were supposed to provide support and protection to the person discriminated against-parents, close family members, employers, and doctors.

The individual with overweight experiences this treatment in the workplace, at home, in school from teachers and students alike, and even from doctors, interns, medical students, nurses, dietitians, and psychologists.

The overweight individual is convinced he deserves the discriminatory and offensive treatment he experiences

Women with overweight are the target of social stigma when it comes to romantic relationships. In a study[47] held in 2007 among 238 students in the U.S., it was found that men are more likely to respond to a singles ad iffrom a woman with normal weight than by a woman with overweight. It was further found that in the case of a woman with overweight, the participants' rate of response was lower when the excess weight was described negatively and included the word "fat" when compared to a more refined description like "full figured."

An additional study[48] held in 2005 examining 554 female students in the U.S. showed that those who avoid dating were heavier than those who dated often or had a regular partner. The researchers calculated and found that the average chance for a woman to be in a healthy romantic relationship decreases with an increase in her weight.

In the workplace the situation is no less dire. In the same survey[49] mentioned earlier and held among 2,249 overweight women, a quarter of them reported weight discrimination in the workplace. Half of them reported feeling as if they have been stigmatized by colleagues and 43% reported being stigmatized by their employer.

Of the overall population with obesity it was found that women were the most vulnerable. A little over a quarter of them reported wrongdoing regarding their weight. The findings of the Rudd Institute at the University of Connecticut show that this discrimination is manifested in not getting hired, being given menial tasks, or outright dismissal on the grounds of not losing weight.

In our day an age, where the Diet Language is the native language, it seems that the rights of an individual with overweight is not respected by anyone.

STIGMA AND DISCRIMINATION BY MEDICAL PROFESSIONALS

Studies that examined the positions and attitudes of medical professionals- doctors, nurses, and dietitians- revealed that the majority of them are bound by negative stereotypes regarding people whose weight does not fit in with standard values. Out of the many studies pointing to this I will mention only one[50] , from 2003, which examined the perceptions of 600 doctors and showed that over half of them agreed that people with overweight can be attributed more negative traits. They are strange, sexually unattractive, and ugly. One third of the doctors agreed with the statement that people with overweight have negative character traits such as lack of willpower, clumsiness, laziness, and unresponsiveness to treatment. Doctors find it difficult to treat a personl with obesity and allot him less time, treating him in a hostile and accusatory manner. And patients sense everything. Indeed, people who suffer from weight discrimination avoid treatment and medical supervision, thus worsening their medical problems. The belief that obesity is a behavioral problem puts the blame and failure on the individual with obesity and increases the negative attitude towards him.

Dietitians, whose job it is to assist the individual with obesity, are no different from the doctors in their attitude towards the obese and obesity. In March 2009, the leading publication for dietitians in the U.S.[51] published an article stating that dietitians are also bound by stigmas judging the individualwith overweight. The study examined the attitudes of nutrition students who may become dietitians about people with overweight and how this affects the treatment decision and the assessment of the patient's health. Over 40% of the students stated they believe that people with overweight are lazy, lack willpower and are inclined to give in to their desires. Most of them agreed that people with obesity have little self-discipline, eat too much, are insecure and have low self-esteem.

What may be the most saddening number: only 2% of the students expressed a positive or neutral approach towards patients with obesity. Studies that examined veteran dietitians reached similar results. They too are not free from feeling prejudice about their patients.

A study[52] held in England and published in August 2013 evaluated the bias towards the obese individual among 1130 students of nutrition, nursing, medicine, and dietetics and attempted to examine the factors that can predict this bias. The results showed that a majority of the students had "fat phobia" and only 1.4% of them displayed a positive or neutral attitude towards the obese population.

THE EFFECTS OF THE STIGMA

Stigma and weight discrimination impact health, employment, social life, and emotions. From a health perspective, studies show a link between the stigma attached to overweight people and the frequency of binges and unhealthy eating. This stigma increases the possibility for developing symptoms of eating disorders (mainly bulimia) and lack of physical activity. Discrimination pushes dieting with the purpose of changing the situation by losing weight. The experience of failing again and again intensifies the stigma as well as the weight gain. A study[53] published in August 2013 which spanned 6,157 participants, showed that those who didn't have obesity at the beginning of the study but experienced weight discrimination were 2.5 more inclined to gain weight than those who had not experienced this type of discrimination after four years of follow up. Those who had obesity when the study began were three times more inclined to stay that way when they experienced this type of discrimination. People who suffer from the negative social attitude towards fat people are in a high state of stress accompanied by an increase in blood pressure. This overall situation leads to neglect and a decrease in the quality of life.

Psychologically, the stigma attached to a person due to his weight causes anxiety, loss of self-esteem, low body image, depression, and suicidal thoughts. All of these distances the person from the social life cycle, creating isolation which alternately causes overeating and attempts at dieting, only to find that weight gain is the only result either way.

Financially, socially, and in the field of employment, the statistics are dire. People with obesity often suffer from low pay, unjust dismissal, unfair and unequal treatment, disciplinary measures, and disrespectful and belittling treatment. The experience of rejection and stigma is met by the individual with obesity in universities, clothing stores, restaurants, and public transport. And the more he weighs, the more he's discriminated against.

According to the Diet Language, the individual with obesity is perceived as the architect of his own disease-eating too much and doing too little. Studies show that the more the "disease" a person suffers from is perceived to be linked to control and self-responsibility, the more anger and resentment it invokes, and the less mercy, help, and empathy receives.

A study examining 66 kinds of diseases and health situations found that the level of a person's personal responsibility over his illness will affect the level of rejection he will experience and the social support he will receive.

Weight discrimination intensifies obesity

WHOSE FAULT IS IT BUT YOUR OWN?

"You're the one who doesn't make any effort and doesn't shut his mouth. You're the one who doesn't exercise enough. You're the one who cheats on your diet. Don't you realize you're about to fail?"

No, these are not the words of his therapist or doctor. Nor the words of his wife who loves him just as he is. These are his own words. He's the one who is furious at himself. He has fully internalized society's expectations of him and he's convinced they're his own. And this is how he walks about the world, guilty guilty, guilty, guilty...

Guilty for not working out today, guilty for eating a little bit more than what's allowed, guilty for not watching himself. Guilty! And here he is abusing himself. And he does it best. His inner critic never rests. I

Then he goes to the doctor and says to him, "Doctor, I know I'm not okay, help me. Give me such a strict diet that I'll have no choice but to follow it." And to his wife he says, "What are you doing with me, can't you see I'm a complete loser? Look at my giant gut. My heaviness and limpness. What do you need a man like that for around the house?" and these are not words said in order to earn some grace and mercy. They come from complete belief that this is what he is. He's guilty and he must pay the price. This is how he goes to work, this is how he raises his children and this is how he talks to his friends.

AN END WHICH IS ALSO A BEGINNING

Pain, any way we look at it, is an inseparable part of life. Some will say it is what gives them meaning, some will say we create it, but no matter how we choose to see it, it exists. Suffering is our reaction to pain, bit it is subjective. It has no rules, boundaries, or formal definitions. It exists because it exists and its essence stems from some confusion between thoughts and reality and from the intense desire for things to be different than they are, without understanding why we don't succeed in making it so. The question is what part we play incausing and holding onto it.

> *Release from suffering requires acknowledging reality*

The Diet Language creates much suffering. The suffering is entailed in the way society defines the individual according to his weight and with his recurring failure in achieving the thinness ideal.

Life lived according to the Diet Language becomes a life full of pain, guilt.

> *"It's not enough to open the window*
> *To see the fields and the river.*
>
> *It's also not enough to not be blind*
> *To see the trees and the flowers.*
> *It's also necessary to not have any philosophy at all.*
> *With philosophy there are no trees, there are only ideas.*
> *There's only each of us, like a wine-cellar.*
> *There's only a shut window and the world outside it;*
> *And a dream of what you could see if you opened the window,*
> *Which is never what you see when you open the window."*[54]

PART TWO: HOW TO BE FREED FROM SUFFERING

THE SALUTOGENIC APPROACH PROMOTING HEALTH AND THE LANGUAGE OF MINDFUL EATING

"Although things are constantly changing, there is no need or option for you to change anything, but only for you to deeply comprehend the way things work. If you delve in deep, you will find that the past has gone and is impossible to change, the future does not exist anywhere but in your expectations in the present, and the present is here with you now. Then you will learn to understand that change is nothing but a philosophical idea."[55]

Every person has a congenital wish to promote their health. This is a key idea in the salutogenic- health focused medical approach. According to this approach, developed by the American-Israeli sociologist Aaron Antonovsky, instead of focusing on illness or identifying risk factors, guilt and fear, the focus must be on health and on identifying the genetic, physical, social, emotional and spiritual factors which encourage it.

According to the salutogenic approach, the motivation to change lies in promoting joy and happiness in life and people have an inner desire and ability to adopt healthy behaviors. According to this approach, we should never stimgatize a person- who is a complex human being with many attributes- because he or she has a certain disease, disability, or any other specific trait. Striving for vitality and health is what leads people to change, not the fear of mortality and morbidity.

Instead of seeing us struggling with symptoms and trying to make them disappear as the cure, we will attempt to transform our relationship with symptoms so the person no longer sees them as symptoms with the assumption that the attempts to make the symptoms disappear increases suffering and does not necessarily promote health.

Body weight is a physical given. Like height, waist circumference, hair color, and sexual orientation. Once body weight becomes a value instead of a measurement, other taglines are attached to it: dangerous, bad, embarrassing. And immediately the need to "banish" it arises. We learn that only a life with no excess weight can be healthy and happy.

Most people believe they are not okay and need to be fixed. They usually feel that they lack willpower, a sense of self-worth, and other traits they believe others possess. They believe they have bad traits like anxiety, negative thoughts, excess weight and painful memories which need to be removed from their lives in order for them to be able to live and move on.

> *Body weight is a physical given. Like height, hair color, and sexual orientation. It does not say anything about my qualities as a person*

These perceptions aggravate two processes:

- Labeling by using negative terms: dysfunctional, maladaptive, irrational, negative. Presumably the person has broken down, and bad elements that must be removed for him to be healthy.In the world of obesity, this is dysfunctional eating, disordered eating, compulsive eating, and being overweight.
- Attempting to replace oreliminate unwanted or unpleasant thoughts, emotions, memories, or situations.

We often perceive ourselves as damaged and in need of fixing if our weight deviates even by a few kilos from what is viewed and valued as legitimate.

What would happen if we saw weight for what it really is, as nothing but a measurement, without the label we have attached to it? If we saw that it is as primarily the result of a genetic array and countless diets that have tried to change this tendency? And what would happen if we add to this the acknowledgement that there is no real guaranteed way to lose weight and keep it off?

If we internalize these ideas we might feel like we have nothing to be ashamed of and no one to hide from. Maybe weight will no longer be the center of our lives. Maybe it will finally stop controlling us once and for all.

A HEALTH FOCUSED APPROACH AND THE LANGUAGE OF MINDFUL EATING

The health focused approach- as opposed to the weight focused approach- is rooted in the world views and treatment approaches particular to populations on the two ends of the Gauss Scale- a curve of normal distribution. On the right end of the curve are people suffering from morbid obesity, what is also called grade two and threeobesity (BMI >35) and on the left end of the curve are those who are extremely thin, who suffer from eating disorders (BMI<18.5). The new approach is based on the "Health at Every Size" (HAES) paradigm.

In many ways the genesis of this movement can be seen in the social-political movements, the SAA (Size Acceptance Approach) movements that arose in the late sixties and raised the banner of acceptance of different shapes and sizes and promoting health to people regardless of their body weight and size. The first of them was founded in 1969 and called the National Association to Aid Fat Americans. It was a nonprofit human rights organization, committed to improving the quality of life of people with obesity, and the rest is history.

Today this approach groups together professionals in the fields of health and education, intellectuals, and social commentators, claiming that focusing on body weight as the indication to improve health and quality of life not only doesn't solve the problem of obesity, but worsens it. The approach is based on acceptance and respect for the natural differences in body shape and size and believes that if we eat pleasurably with regard to our natural codes of hunger and satiation and live an active life, we will reach the body weight we are naturally meant to have. This does not mean a drastic change will occur our in body weight and we'll be thin within the beauty ideal or the standard BMI measures, but we will certainly improve our physical and mental health.

> *Every person has a set-point in which he was meant to be and it does not necessarily match BMI measures*

The health focused approach bases itself on a combination of the humanist organist perception and the salutogenic model of health developed by Aaron Antonovsky[56]. The organistic perceptions are perceptions that see the behavior of the living organism and its traits as a whole being, in which there are interactions between the complete organism and its components and between the components themselves. While the humanistic perceptions wish to focus on the issue of realizing and expanding humankind's humanity and developing its latent human resources towards creation and development.

The salutogenic model (source of health) which completes the philosophical basis for the health focused approach assumes that we cannot categorize people dichotomically as healthy or sick. It is possible to distinguish people who are in a state of "ease" on one end of the scale and those who are in a state of "disease" on the other end of it, and the different levels between them.

The question is not what causes some disease or other but what explains the motion towards the healthy end of the ease-disease scale. If the pathogenic model focuses on what causes diseases, the salutogenic model has turned the focus to an overall view of the person and finding the active factors that promote his health.

Antonovsky, who developed the salutogenic approach, is spiritually close to the Buddhist approach, which states that human life is filled with hardship, stress, and suffering whether we like it or not, and the same goes for disease risk factors. "It is better to focus on resources and the ability to create health than focus on the risks and morbidity," he said.

Based on this world view, Antonovsky contemplated the issue "How do people stay healthy?" Which lead to the development of another key phrase: "a sense of coherence." The sense of coherence is thought to be an internal coping resource which helps the individual stand up and cope in a positive way with stressful situations, thus helping maintain mental and physical health.

The sense of coherence, according to Antonovsky, is A global orientation which expresses the range in which the individual has a strong and flexible sense of security (or a sense of trust) and the stimuli that arise from his internal and external environment, during life are understandable, predictable and reasonable.

The sense of coherence consists of three key elements: meaningfulness, comprehensibility, and manageability.

Meaningfulness: The emotional element of the sense of coherence is the extent to which a person feels there is meaning to life, even when unpleasant events or situations occur such as being fired, suffering disease, or the death of a relative. In these situations, a person with a high tendency towards meaningfulness will consciously regard these stressful events as challenges and a means to grow, even if he experiences sorrow. Small everyday pressures of life, in the workplace, and the family will also be perceived by a person with a high tendency for meaningfulness as a challenge, and not a heavy burden. Antonovsky claims that a higher sense of meaning will also enable understanding the "free" side of life. Thus, the person's ability to participate in shaping his life and his designation, and the awareness that a person has some control over his life.

Comprehensibility: The cognitive element of the sense of coherence is the extent to which the person perceives the world and the stress, coping, demands, and stimuli he experiences in his life as having cognitive significance. This is the person's ability to create "cognitive order," thus perceiving the world as a place that has inner order and a certain ability to predict what is to come (the sun rises every day and it also sets) and apply that order to his internal and external world. The acquired information will then be orderly, consistent, structured, and comprehensible instead of chaotic, disordered, incidental, and incomprehensible. A person with a high sense of comprehensibility will believe that when the future comes (both immediate and distant) it will be predictable, or in case of surprise,logical consequences with a steady and orderly inner structure will still be able to be made.

Manageability: the behavioral element of the sense of coherence is examined by the extent in which the person has enough resources to cope with the world and life's demands. A person with a high sense of manageability will feel as if he has enough tools at hand to manage his life and meet the demands set by internal and external stimuli. This person will not feel as if he is the victim of a situation and will see his life as pretty fair. The coping resources can be internal, or they can also be a "legitimate other" like partners, friends, God, culture, and anything else the person has established trust in.

The salutogenic model allows the problem of obesity to be looked at from a new point of view: not a battle with weight gain and not an endless attempt to make it disappear so we can have what we think is a full and healthy life. The question driving those who believe in this approach is: how do we help people find their health promoting points of strength with their existing weight? My life doesn't begin after losing weight and does not entail it. It is here and now, in the present, about me as a complete person, whose weight is just a small part of. It is possible to live a healthy and complete life at any body weight (again, this does not mean "let's be fat", but it does mean that we put aside the doomed to fail struggle with weight and try to promote a full, healthy life with our existing weight).

The shift from a weight focused approach to a health focused approach is the shift from one philosophical approach to another. From an approach that fights weight gain and obesity to an approach that focuses on promoting health with weight.

The health focused approach is based on a number of principles:

- The endless preoccupation with weight and diets intensifies the obesity problem, disrupts eating habits and peoples' relationship with their bodies.
- A natural, legitimate difference in body shape and weight exists- real people come in all shapes and sizes.
- Every person has their own set-point.
- Happiness has no weight.
- Eating with attention to hunger and satiation, free of restriction, will lead to a healthy body weight and keep it stable.
- You don't have to be thin to be healthy, but those at the ends of the weight scale are at risk and must be treated.

According to this approach, the treatment's success relies on a combination of physiological measures like blood pressure, blood lipids (blood fats) and blood sugar level with psychological measures like feelings that accompany eating, eating behaviors, self-esteem, depression, body image, and anxiety.

The eating language that accompanies the health focused approach is the language of intuitive eating, or by its other name- Mindful Eating.

The Mindful Eating language, which relies on the body's inner authority and its subjective signals of hunger and satiation, can lead a person to healthy eating behaviors. It relies on unique human nature. Each and every one of us is endowed with a variety of needs, desires and appetites. Therefore, every person can gauge by his own personal scale of hunger and satiation if he's hungry, what he is hungry for, when he would like to eat and how much.

If we are mindful of personal hunger and satiation, we will reach the body weight we were genetically meant to be. This weight is not necessarily the weight we would like to be, but it is surely the weight we can be. A weight at which we will live a full, healthy life.

Studies show that adopting the Mindful Eating language leads to improvement in physiological measures (like blood pressure and blood lipid level) in healthy behavior (physical activity, healthy eating) and in psychological measures that are expressed in mood, self-confidence, and body image even with no weight loss.

- *Every person is entitled and deserves to enjoy the food he eats and eat to satiation*
- *The body can and should be respected and loved even if it does not fit into the "thin model"*
- *Not all people were meant to be thin due to our genetic traits*
- *Body weight is not a measure of success or failure*
- *Weight is not a measure of health*
- *Happiness has no weight*

NOT ANOTHER DIET

"So you really mean that you don't know how to help me lose weight and stay thin?"

"Yes," I replied, my heart pounding.

"And you want me to stay fat?"

"No, I don't want you to stay fat at all, but I know that my attempts to help you lose weight will only hurt you and your body, which always eventually finds its way back up.I can't sell you the illusion and I can't put you back into the diet cycle." "Well if you ensure that I stay fat, what do I even need you for?" she replied.

I sensed her outrage at me for not being able to promise her what she wants to hear so badly. Because what does she care about hunger and satiation, Mindful Eating, and self-acceptance? All these terms look great on paper, but when you want to go on dates or shop for clothes they become faded words that have no meaning.

"It's true," she said. "My head is full of noise, thoughts of what is forbidden and allowed, right, wrong, how much I ate, why and when, what I have to do to burn off all the calories I ate...all that is true. I'm really tired, tired of the attempts and failures but mainly of the guilt and fear that keeps calling me 'fat, fat, fat.' "

I look at her blue eyes, her flowing hair, her carefully done nails and her pretty dress, hiding remarkably sexy curves, And I wonder, "Does she really not see how attractive she is?" I'm not trying to convince her of her value, and not trying to convince her to be treated by me, but I say to her, "It's true, Sigal. I understand you. It's difficult to hear what you don't want to hear. And it's even more difficult to start a process of therapy that does not ensure conquering the dream you have been waiting for. But..." I took a deep breath. "I can offer you a complete, different world. Where you don't count, you don't measure; you don't feel guilt...a world of choice, freedom, free to feel real pleasure from eating and a bit of pleasure from that self that we are so used to being angry with. I know this is not what you wish for, but your old shoes are already torn. Isn't it time to stop?

She looks at me...having a hard time letting go...not moving from her chair. Sneaking a look into my eyes, looking me up and down and over again, she finally says, "You don't understand anything...you're thin. You just don't get it."

"What if I was fat?" I reply, "What would you have said then? That I'm trying to justify my weight? Once we give meaning to what we weigh, it has meaning. But what is this scale other than a metal object? What is it other than a cold object we have given the power to run our lives? That determines whether we feel beautiful or not, if we eat a full meal today or make do with a piece of light bread, if we have to go to the gym or if we're allowed to go shopping?"

She finally looked at me. She seemed a bit surprised. "So you understand a little bit," she said. I smiled. I sensed the ice had been broken. And not because I'm fat or thin or before a diet or after it, but because I understand exactly what she understands: That she has become a slave to these numbers that hurt her day in and day out. That she has long been a slave to her body instead of its master. And she smiled. Not because the loop she is caught in has been opened, but mainly because she was feeling as if she was sitting in the right chair.

OPTIMISM IS THE NAME OF THE GAME

"What is the path?
Joshu asked (his teacher) Nansen: `What is the path'?
Nansen said: `It is the thought of the everyday life'.
Joshu asked: `You have to aim for it, don't you'?
Nansen said: `Once you aimed for it, you have already missed it'.
Joshu asked: `If I don't aim for it, how can I know it is the path'?
Nansen said: `The path has nothing to do with knowing or not knowing. Knowing is a blind perception. Not knowing is simply unreceptiveness. If you reach the path not aimed for, it is like the empty space, absolutely clear. You cannot force it'.
Hearing these words, Joshu was enlightened.[57] "

Einstein said that we cannot solve problems with the same mind that created them. Then what do we expect when we continue trying to solve weight problems with the same language that has created them? True, it is difficult to part with the Diet Language, especially in light of the fact that most people speak it. Even so, this process brings great relief, release from suffering, and yes, a fuller, healthier, more livable life. It feels like an exit from slavery to freedom.

This path does not:

- Deal with teaching alternative techniques whose goal is weight loss
- Measure success in kilograms
- Provide techniques to control eating or weight
- Deal with the question of "why." Why did you eat? Why did you gain weight? Why did you eat this and not that? How much? Where?

This path, in a positive way:

- Doubts what we think is the only truth and focuses on the way in which we are the architects of what we see and know in accordance to what we want to see and know
- Frees us from the Diet Language
- Normalizes the relationship with the body and eating so they will no longer be a symptom that manages life
- Focuses on the acceptance of given weight as a part of life. Acceptance which enables a full life led by peoples' true values with their existing body weight and not necessarily without it.
- Looks at the "War on Fat" and the diet and thinness industry with a critical eye.
- Uses mindfulness and acceptance techniques
- Clarifies that all eating whose overt or covert objective is weight loss leads to a disruption of eating and the relationship with the body.
- Leads to one of the three following options: maintaining weight, slimming down to the individual's unique set-point, or gaining weight to the set-point.
- Leads to a full and healthy life at every body shape and size. Real people come in all sizes.

MINDFULNESS- THE WAY TO BE

"Someone who heard my poem said to me: What's new about this?
Everyone knows that a flower is a flower and a tree is a tree.
But I replied: Not everyone, no one.
Everyone loves flowers because they are beautiful, and I'm different.
Everyone loves the trees because they are green and give shade, but not I.
I love the flowers because they are flowers, openly.
I love the trees because they are trees, without thought."[58]

Mindfulness, a life approach studied in the East for hundreds of years, started making its way into the West in the 1980's. Jon Kabat Zin is considered the first to use mindfulness in a non-religious way to help patients in hospitals handle chronic pain. In recent years mindfulness is beginning to be implemented in other fields of therapy in reducing episodes of depression, reducing anxiety symptoms, reducing chronic pain, reducing binge eating, and providing tools for handling stress.

Mindfulness is a reasonable approach to life. It means paying attention to the mind in the present moment in a way which allows us to experience things without judging them or interpreting them. This is the ability to notice thoughts, feelings, and emotions that arise at a given moment, whether external or internal, without adhering to criticism, judgment, or the desire for things to be different than what they are. This does not mean that you have to love things as they are. This process of observation enables acceptance of internal experiences and minimization of avoidances.

Mindfulness does not instruct you what to do, but at any moment, it enables and opens the door to choose the best thing to do.

Mindfulness affects cognitive and behavioral reactions which are refined when we succeed in being present in the now. Adopting these qualities highly affects interpersonal and intrapersonal relationships.

Using it endows the person with the ability to express and feel generosity, empathy, gratitude, gentleness, love and kindness. These emotional reactions promote the ability to see clearly and be more present in the here and now.

Mindfulness is a way of knowing.

LACK OF MINDFULNESS

The mindfulness techniques are skills which require practice. Many people are distracted on a daily basis by countless situations. As a result of this they can become lost, full of anxiety, disappointed and not really understand what happened and why the situation didn't occur as they had hoped. Here are some situations in which we might find ourselves losing our mindful way:

- When getting lost or missing turn while driving or hiking.

- During a conversation in which we suddenly find we don't understand what people are talking about.

- When watching a movie andwe find ourselves busy and preoccupied with what we'll buy for dinner when the movie's over.

- During a conversation in which we plan what we're going to say before our partner is done talking.

- While reading a book andbeing preoccupied at the same time with an event that was discussed on the news After placing the book on the shelf and we don't recall where we put it.

- We are so busy with our plans during a shower that when we get out we can't recall if we washed our hair.

- While eating we're so busy counting calories and calculating how much we're allowed to eat until the end of the day that we have no idea what we're eating and what we're feeling- are we full?

You're probably asking, "What so wrong with that? Must we always be attentive and connected to every single moment? Is it not possible that these moments of disconnecting from the here and now may actually be good?" Of course. There is no question about the fact that it is sometimes good and even useful to not be present in the now, but this disconnection may sometimes be harmful and destructive.

Here's an exercise that demonstrates what I mean: make yourself a cup of tea and follow the steps of preparation.

- Boil water
- Take a teabag and put it in the cup
- Add sugar
- Pour the water over the bag
- Stir
- Let the bag sink into the water
- Take the bag out
- Add a teaspoon of sugar
- Stir again
- Take the cup of tea in your hand
- Wrap your hands around it
- Feel the heat of the cup
- What do you feel?
- Bring the cup to your lips
- Feel the steam on your face
- Blow on the tea
- Smell the tea

- Take a long sip
- Did it burn your mouth?
- Is it hot?
- Nice and warm?
- What does it taste like?

What did you feel? What did you see? What did you discover while following the steps to their every detail?

MINDFULNESS IS:

- Observing mental processes without attraction or rejection. Observing all aspects of the experience without developing a preference to some occurrence or other. When a pleasant thought appears, we will continue to observe it without desiring it to continue existing, and we won't try to banish an unpleasant thought.
- The ability to be in full attention without classifying the experience as pleasant or pleasurable, painful or unpleasant, and without the activity that links it to other familiar experiences.
- The ability to experience things without needing to stimulate other mental functions but maintaining attention itself with openness, curiosity, and flexibility that allows the experience to take place to its full extent.
- A path which requires concentration, attention, ignoring what is desired and focusing on what exists and is based on the person deciding where and how he turns his attention.
- A path which allows us to discover transience- a thought followed by another one, a feeling followed by another feeling. They come and they go.

- A path that helps us see the process in which the present is created, knowing the truth, renouncing the illusion.
- Simply observing, without a goal or purpose.

The use of mindfulness opens and enables points of view that are usually inaccessible to us, because we operate automatically in our daily routine. The use of mindfulness allows us:

- The ability to be fully present in the here and now.
- To free ourselves from previous stipulations and from automatic rules or strict patterns that often prevent us from acting and living in accordance with our true values.
- To clear the mind of what has accumulated in it, to deconstruct existing mental structures and create a mental space clear of prejudice. That is to say: clearing the mind of prejudice, stigmas, criticism and judgment that do not allow us an unbiased presense in what is taking place.
- To be able to experience unpleasant thoughts and feelings safely, to open the door to those thoughts and feelings that we usually tried to run from.
- To be aware of the experiences we avoid.
- To connect to ourselves, to others, and to the world around us.
- To increase our self-awareness.
- To create the distance which allows us to observe our thoughts, to realize our thoughts and ourselves are not one.
- To have a wider, more open view.

- To know that everything changes. Thoughts and feelings come and go, like shifts in the weather do. Everything is transient.
- To be able to observe ourselves from above while we're participating in an event or undergoing a certain experience. In this way our automatic involvement in the situation is avoided and we are able to reach balance.
- To experience peace, a calm that appears out of nowhere. An ease that in many tumultuous situations gives us a sense that it is okay as it is. A feeling that prevents fighting, fleeing, or avoiding.
- To be accepting and compassionate towards ourselves.
- To be without judgment- to observe and watch without assessing and cataloging our experiences. These are skills that are difficult to adapt to since our automatic tendency is to judge and asses things as good or bad. Judgment binds our vision and narrows it. It causes loss of information and experiences. Lack of judgment allows a more open, flexible and authentic view of the world.
- To be without a goal- the ability to not adhere or grasp onto certain goals since they cause us to miss the joy of the here and now and make us miss other achievements that were not included in our goals in the first place. For instance, if we eat a piece of cake and while we eat it we are constantly anxious of the weight we might gain or fearing the cholesterol within it, we will not be able to take any pleasure in eating the cake and miss the point of eating it. Or if, for instance, someone starts exercising

regularly because he fantasizes about losing weight but doesn't lose a significant amount of it,, he might retire from physical activity, even if it makes him feel better, because it supposedly didn't help him achieve his goal.

- To be patient- this is the ability to allow things to develop at their own pace and in their own time by understanding and accepting that different people have different rhythms and everything that happens in it has its own time.

- To have trust- a sense of security and confidence in yourself, in others, and in the ability of processes to develop.

- The ability to let go- this is the rational ability to not hold on, not to adhere to feelings, thoughts and experiences. This is the ability not to adhere to myself and to the world. It is the ability to understand and recognize the temporary nature of all things and not grasp onto feelings, thoughts, things, or other beings.

The use of mindfulness seems to be as a tool that leads to some longed for change. A tool that brings forth some exciting enlightenment and promises various achievements. But actually it is not a tool at all, but a way to be. Mindfulness is a way of life which requires much practice. And practice, by nature, is not very exciting.

Indeed, those who intend to get to know mindfulness fully should put aside their expectations for a magical transformation. Lower expectations will allow the practice to be experienced more precisely, minute to minute.

People, by nature, are goal and achievement oriented. That is why the mindfulness technique is difficult to learn and practice without a defined purpose. The question of "What am I getting out of this?" is always there. But it is important to understand that grasping on to targets is one of the roots of suffering. If we walked a certain path to reach certain goals, and didn't reach them- our disappointment is self-fulfilling. Specifically, if a person enters the process of treating the language of eating with weight loss at the head of his hopes- disappointment is ready and waiting. Because here he is undergoing an amazing process of language transformation. His eating changes and becomes healthier, the binge eating disappears, and he's even more at peace with his body, but the anticipated weight loss refuses to come and so his goal crumbles before he reaches it.

I invite you to take a look into a world where judgments, criticism, and planning towards achievements and goals have a different place than the one we've been accustomed to. This does not mean they are absent, but they are given a different ascription.

A few more summation points:
- Mindfulness is not an invitation to part from feelings- it allows us to be in control of them and contain a spectrum of emotions.
- Mindfulness is not an invitation to disconnect from life- it connects the person to others and helps him be connected to his own being.
- Mindfulness is not a quest for ultimate happiness- it helps us accept the full range of emotions instead of grasping onto only to the pleasant ones.
- Mindfulness is not an escape from pain- it helps make room also for pain-and decreases it as a result. Mindfulness is not a religious conversion; it supports us and aids our efforts in any emotional and spiritual tradition.
- Training for mindfulness is nothing interesting or exciting- it requires practice.
- Knowing means not knowing in the observation process.

- There is no right and wrong.
- Knowing means just being.
- Right observation will lead to right action.
- Observation is a state of mind which must be maintained within life and not outside of them.
- An empty mind helps see thoughts clearly.

MINDFULNESS IN EVERYDAY LIFE

So how does this all actually work? At the base of all mindfulness exercises is the instruction: notice X. X could be anything that exists in the here and now, a thought, a feeling, a memory, or anything that we see, hear, touch, taste, and smell. That same X can be a gaze out the window, the sensation of hot water in the shower, the taste of a piece of chocolate in your mouth, a picture of the lungs as air is breathed into them, the noise you hear from the next room and the car when you start the engine. In most mindfulness exercises we are asked:

- To pay attention
- Let thoughts and feelings be- make room for them
- Observe the thoughts that come and go
- Let them go

BEFORE YOU ARE THREE EXAMPLES OF EXERCISES FOR YOU TO EXPERIENCE AND GET A SENSE OF:

A mindfulness exercise whose purpose is to focus on us and our ability to connect to the environment we are in:

- Stop for a moment.
- Look around you and note five things you can see.
- Listen closely and note five things you can hear.
- Note five things you can feel that are in contact with your body (the strap of your watch, your feet on the floor, the air on your face).
- Do all these things- stop, look, listen, and notice- simultaneously.

A mindfulness exercise whose purpose is listening to breathing and thoughts:

- Take ten deep breaths.
- Focus on the breath and the air coming out until the lungs are completely empty, only then allow them to fill themselves.
- Note the sensation of the lungs emptying.
- Note the process of their filling up.
- Note the rib cage rising and falling.
- Note the gentle raising of the shoulders and their drop.
- See if you can let thoughts come and go as if they were cars passing on the street outside your house.
- Expand your attention and simultaneously note your breathing, your body.
- Look around the room and note what you see, hear, smell, and feel, what you touch.

A mindfulness exercise whose purpose is to fully focus on the body's sensations in the present moment:

To begin, sit in a quiet, comfortable place. Turn off all

interrupting noises. Take a few deep, long breaths and close your eyes. Use your imagination and picture a narrow ring, lit in white, hanging over your head like a halo. During the course of the exercise this ring will slide down your body and allow you to notice the different physical sensations. Go on breathing deeply with your eyes closed. Keep seeing the white light as a halo over your heads and note every physical sensation in your body. Anything you feel is okay.

- Notice the halo slowly sliding down your head. Touching the tips of your ears, eyes, and nose. While this is happening, note your sensations.
- See the halo sliding down towards the nose. It touches your cheeks, your mouth. Note your physical sensations.
- Note the sensations on the back of your head as well.
- Note the sensations on your tongue, your teeth.
- Keep on following the ring of light in your imagination. It continues sliding down your neck. Note the tonus of the muscles in the front and back of it.
- And the ring keeps on moving. Here it is at your shoulders.
- Note the sensations that arise there: in your shoulders, upper back, upper arms, and chest.
- The ring continues its journey. Here it is on the arms, the elbows, the hands and the fingers. Note every sensation and feeling that passes through your body, the tension that is created everywhere.
- And the ring moves on and here it is at the lower half of your body. Your stomach, your upper legs.
- Note the sensations at the front of the body

and at the back.

- Go on following the ring until it touches your feet and try to experience every single moment. Every physical sensation that passes through your body.

And now, when the ring touches the floor and fades away, take a number of deep breaths and, at your own pace, open your eyes.

Imagine, if you will, a camera. Place it so the lens is looking over your head or at the point where you believe you mind is located. From this moment, each time you push the record button on your camera, it will capture the existing moments one after the other. It will do this as long as you push the record button. It will be very much in the present moment and its main advantage will be that it films exactly what it sees. Without any judgment, criticism, or opinion. The pictures reflect exactly what is happening under one condition: You must remember to push the record button. To be allowed to be in that present moment, with full attention to everything that is happening. We must want to see.

MINDFUL IN EATING

Most peoples' eating is governed by millions of beliefs and stigmas, fear, and guilt. Anything we eat is measured, counted, compared to what was eaten yesterday, what should have been eaten, what the other person has eaten and what we think we will eat tomorrow. Because of this, any eating that does not comply with the rules is harshly judged. It is difficult to observe, to see, to acknowledge. Mostly because of the difficulty and anxiety of "what will be discovered, what we will discover and how guilty we'll feel." Because of this, many leave eating as it is: automatic and habitual. We have a hard time observing it. We choose to eat on autopilot. But we must dare and want to see. We must have the courage to push the record button on the camera. We must make a decision and ready ourselves internally to dare, discover, and see (even if it is scary).

I'll emphasize again: while you are in the process of acquiring "Mindful Eating" language I am not inviting you to do the usual meditation exercises. I am also not inviting you to devote a certain amount of time every day to the observation process. I want to be practical and realistic. It is difficult today to ask most people to stop the race and make time for fifteen minutes of meditation and observation every day. Although this is recommended, I assume for most of us it is still impossible.

I will try to give you the ability to observe the mind during life and not by disconnecting from it. I will not search for perfect but focus on the whole. On what you can do at any given moment. Mindfulness can be attained when you are eating, getting up, talking, watching television. And you can attain Mindful Eating at any moment that has to do with eating.

We won't wait for special moments when we are eating alone, but try to be attentive to our eating regularly, on a daily basis. Whenever it begins, occurs, ends. We will listen to our bodies, our thoughts, our hunger, fullness, pleasure. And this does not mean counting, measuring, weighing, fearing. Because if we are to witness eating, we will do so from the point of view of the observer, free of criticism and comparison. This mindfulness, once you discover it, will accompany you forever. Without judgment and expectations and with a wish to be present and attentive to your body's needs, to flavor, joy, hunger, and satiation. This mindfulness will forever be part of the eating experience.

SECULAR MINDFULNESS TECHNIQUES

In the following I will present to you useful mindfulness techniques that can accompany you in your everyday life and be good for eating as well as other fields of life, without you needing to anchor yourselves in meditation sessions.

- **The three minute mindfulness**

This techniques helps us notice if we're mindful and returns us to mindfulness if we have grown far from it. Whether we are sitting at our desk at work, and whether you're at the bus station or just in the TV room, you can practice three minute mindfulness. There is no need to disconnect yourself from the world, only to try and develop maximum attention as the world rushes noisily by. Pay attention to the thoughts, emotions and sensations you feel in the here and now. Let them be, and accept them. Don't try to push them aside or avoid them. Make room for them. Acknowledge them. Now, fully listen to your breaths. Notice them. Their entry, their exit. Now take a minute to shift your attention to other parts of your body. Recognize them. Accept all that is present and existing in this moment.

- **Mindfulness with use of your surroundings**

Using signals from your surroundings can remind us of the need for mindfulness and empower you in the present.

When the phone rings, instead of rushing to pick it up, stop for a minute, smile, breathe. Let the phone ring a bit more before you rush to answer it. Follow the ringing. Follow yourselves picking it up. Remind yourselves to be open and receptive to any phone call, regardless of its content.

You can be similarly attentive to the dog barking in the yard, the siren of an ambulance, the scent of a cake baking in the oven, to knocks at your door. You can basically make use of any signal from your surroundings to remind you and allow you to be mindful in the moment.

- **Senses- sound**

Listen carefully to background noises. Try to distinguish each particular sound. Listen to the sound of raindrops on the roof, of passing cars, of your neighbor's radio and the music it's playing, of the nearby house's AC motor, of birds and crickets chirping, of footsteps on a silent street in the middle of the night. You can listen to a specific sound or to the range of sounds. Most importantly: listen. You can stick with a certain sound for a few minutes and then deliberately divert your attention and listen to a different sound. This practice will create the distinction between hearing and listening.

- **Senses- smell**

Try following a certain scent. Or try to generally understand what scents you usually enjoy. Notice how the scent enters your nostrils and how the breath rises and falls following it. Note how you react to different types of scents and the different sensations these scents awake within us. Try to notice just the scent, without categorizing it.

MINDFULNESS AND THE LANGUAGE OF EATING

Mindfulness has a key role in changing the language of eating and parting from the Diet Language.

By using it,

- We will see and acknowledge the Diet Language as that which governs our eating. The thoughts, feelings, rules, and beliefs it has created which dictate what we eat, when, how much, and why and how we feel before eating during it and after it. It will allow us to see how this language disrupts our eating, hurts the "self", causes binge eating and sometimes even makes us gain weight.

- We will learn to let go of the Diet Language, to part from it.
- We will learn to listen to the needs of our body free of prejudice, guilt, and fear.
- We will learn to recognize the authentic and individual hunger and satiation signals, unique to each one of us. We will learn not to slide into automatic mode in managing our eating.
- We will allow ourselves choice. From nonjudgmental observation we will be able to choose what to eat, how much, and how. And not because we were told to choose, but because we chose to.

In summation: mindfulness is based on four foundations:

acceptance, being in the here and now, acquiring the position of the observing self and the ability to let go. The four of these together will be used by us in our path to letting go of the Diet Language and acquiring the language of Mindful Eating.

CONTROL IS THE PROBLEM- ACCEPTANCE IS THE SOLUTION

"There being injustice is like there being death.
I would never take a step to change
What they call the the world's injustice.
A thousand steps taken for that
Would only be a thousand steps.
I accept injustice like I accept a stone not being a perfect circle,
And a cork tree not growing into a pine or an oak.
I cut an orange in two, and the two parts can't be equal.
Which one was I unjust to — I, who am going to eat them
both?"[59]

Acceptance is the ability to allow thoughts, feelings and situations be as they are, whether they are painful or pleasant. Acceptance is the ability to make room for them, to let go of fighting them and allow them to be as they are. Acceptance is the ability to be fully open, with no defenses and no rigidity and open the door even to unwanted and painful experiences. Acceptance helps us work towards a healthy, full life and towards realizing everyone's individual values.

When to use it- when the struggle with avoidant thoughts and behaviors becomes an obstacle for fully realizing our values.

What turns pain into suffering is our struggle with it and our difficulty to accept it. The belief is that in order to live well we must get rid of pain. But pain is a part of life.

In our day to day life, whenever we experience a problem, we immediately try to solve it. Whenever we encounter pain, we try to extricate ourselves from it. There are situations in which this tendency helps. If we're cold, we put on a sweater. If we have a headache, we take an aspirin. A problem arises and we find a solution for it. But this method of coping is incompatible with coping with our thoughts and feelings.

Acceptance is opening a door to the existence of feelings, emotions, urges, passions, thoughts, and situations that -even if they are difficult and cause suffering- are still an inseparable part of human existence.

The acceptance process is difficult but it actually includes what exists in life anyway, even if we don't want it. To accept things as they are does not mean to want them or to make friends with them but to see them as a part of life, to observe them, talk to them, see them.

We can simply accept our body weight, even if it's "over" weight. Not because it's better to be fat, but because there is no way to ensure permanent, long-term weight loss. Once we stop struggling with ourselves, we can be free to really improve our lives. Life is no longer managed by fear, anxiety, avoidance, and rigid adherenceto rules and begins being managed by free choice.

Acceptance is not a technique but a process, consisting of four interconnected stages:

- Accepting reality- giving up ignorance, the pursuit of pleasure and the suppression of pain. This process includes seeing the diet industry and the processes of medicalization and the politics of obesity as it truly is, understanding not everyone can be thin or has to be thin in order to be healthy, and that no real solution exists for obesity.
- Accepting the body and accepting the legitimate difference in shape and size between people.
- Letting go of the Diet Language- parting from the language of control.
- Acquiring the language of Mindful Eating- a language of freedom and choice.

> *It is easier to adapt our expectations to reality than to force reality to fit our expectations*

FACTS THAT WE MUST ACCEPT IN ORDER TO BE ABLE TO PART WITH THE DIET LANGUAGE

Accepting reality is no easy feat. In order to acquire the language of Mindful Eating and improve our lives, there are a number of facts that we must acknowledge. Here are some of them:

- Weight is not the product of choice or decision and is not the result of willpower.
- There is no feasible way to lose weight and keep it off over the years.
- Anobsessive preoccupation with body weight and trying to it hurts both our emotional and physical health.
- The Diet Language is a tyrannical, hurtful language which disrupts eating and our relationship with our body.
- The younger our preoccupation with body weight starts, the more it will disrupt the healthy growing process, disrupt eating habits, and cause weight gain over the set-point.
- Avoiding certain foods intensifies binge eating and loss of control over eating.
- A diet- any diet, even those masquerading as lifestyle changers- eventually cause weight gain.
- The use of scales is harmful.
- Happiness has no weight.
- Life is here and now. Not tomorrow. Not later. Not "When I'll be thin."

- Mindful Eating is eating that is guided by codes of hunger and satiation and not by rules which instruct us what to eat, how much, and when.

- Every one of us has natural, personal codes of hunger and satiation.

- Only our body can say what is right to eat, how much, and when.

- Healthy eating is varied eating.

- Pleasure from eating is essential to Mindful Eating.

- Preoccupation with body weight and dieting is often a cover for dealing with emotional situations like loneliness, anxiety, and trauma.

- Every one of us has a set-point which we were genetically meant to be at.

- There is a natural difference between people in their body shape and size- real people come in all sizes.

- Physical activity is an essential part of a healthy life. It is not merely a weight loss tool.

- The diet industry is run by economic interests.

- Weight gain is not a result of caloric balance.

- Weight discrimination exists.

- Weight discrimination increases obesity.

- Obesity is not a disease of kilograms but of malfunctioning fat cells.

- Weight is not a measure of health. You don't have to be thin to be healthy.

- If guilt and shame, intimidation and discrimination could cure obesity, there would be no obese people.

> Suffering stems from wanting the reality to be different
> than what it actually is. Relief stems from accepting
> reality as it is

AND SHE DIDN'T EVEN START TO LOSE WEIGHT YET

It was amazing. There is no doubt she is fat. There is also no doubt that she's convinced that it's all because of her weight, but there is also no doubt that all she did was put on some makeup and get a haircut and hold her head up a bit higher and everyone said to her "Michal, you look great, what did you do?" when in reality she had not done anything yet. She was only planning to undergo gastric sleeve surgery. But something within her let go of the rigid mindset that was destroying her life. One that demanded everything has to go her way, under her watchful gaze, and fit into her one-dimensional vision.And thus her emotional walls began breaking open like those of Jericho.

She has been locked behind them for years. Feeling rejected and undesirable. And she'll show the world her worth, no matter her weight. And she'll show the world she's right. For 22 years out of the 32 she's lived she has been feeling lonely and has an intense need to be seen for who she is and what she is. It's not really her weight, it was just the cover for her inability to relinquish control of everything. And it seems to me that she's beginning to find it. And here her neighbor is smiling at her. A schoolmate even complemented her and took her out for coffee. And she hasn't even lost any weight yet.

BEING PRESENT - CONNECTED TO HERE AND NOW

"Let's only care about the place where we are.
There's beauty enough in being here and not anywhere else.
If there's someone beyond the curve in the road,
Let them worry about what's past the curve in the road,
That's what the road is to them."*

To be in the here and now, to be in the present, fully acknowledging the given moment without escaping or getting lost in thoughts or feelings even if we sense, see, and feel pain.

The purpose - to promote an aware consciousness of experiences occurring in the moment. Gathering information which gives us the choice between changing and maintaining behavior. Being fully engaged in the experience of creating the moment so it can be intensified and realized.

The method - noticing what is happening in the here and now. Distinguishing attention and thought, and noticing the internal world and the external world at once.

When to use it - when we are fully preoccupied with the past and the future. When we are operating on autopilot.

When we loyally adhere to speak the Diet Language we live in the past and future simultaneously. The ability to focus full, nonjudgmental attention on the present, internal as well as external, is a substantial part of the process of acquiring the language of Mindful Eating. The present is the only time that actually exists. And that's the magic of it. Discovering what is coming to be in this exact moment. And it is what it is, in this very moment.

---

* Alberto Caeiro

The ability to be in the here and now is connected to the core of mindfulness. It is always easier to run out and disconnect. To run to thoughts about the past or the future. To cruise on autopilot. Connecting to the here and now means being flexible in the ability to bring our full consciousness to the present moment and not run away to thoughts and fantasies. The more we succeed in being fully aware of our present experiences and minimize our drifting into the future or the past, the more efficient we can be and lead a fuller, richer life.

> *We spend most of our lives longing for the past, planning and fearing the future, and not living in the now. But the past is past, and who can predict the future?*

I AM NOT MY THOUGHT –
COGNITIVE DEFUSION

"I don't know what I feel or what I want to feel. I don't know what to think or what I am."[80]

Cognitive defusion is parting from thoughts in a way which allows them to come and go instead of latching on to them.

- It is the ability to step away
- To observe thoughts instead of be in them
- To notice thoughts and not get caught up in them
- To allow thoughts to come and go instead of grasping on to them or being grasped by them.

The purpose - to see the nature of thoughts, to understand that they are in fact more or less just words and images, and to react to them. To see to what extent they help or harm.

The method - to notice the thought process, to learn in an experiential manner that thoughts don't have to control behavior.

When to use it - when thoughts, emotions or situations stand in the way of our well-being, of realizing our values.

A thought is a group of words which we endow with meaning. We are convinced that our thoughts define us and that they are reality. We tend to believe them, cling to them, and live by them. But reality is not thoughts. Reality is what there is. It exists.

Cognitive defusion is meant to counteract cognitive fusion, the mind's tendency to cling to objects (internal or external) and bind to them.

Many exercises are intended to do so by diverting attention from the content of the thought to other aspects of it, like its visual form when it's written or the sound of its words when spoken.

For instance, if we repeat a certain word aloud a number of times, familiar to us as it may be, it loses its literal meaning and is perceived, for a brief moment, almost as if it were a word in a foreign language or just a meaningless sound. Other exercises try to achieve a similar effect with writing, by observing the thought process itself, and by using humor.

The presumption is that an ability to part from our thoughts will lessen the need to fight them and increase the ability to divert energy and time towards creating a fuller life.

This can be done in three principal ways:
1. Observing our thoughts
2. Noting the efficiency of our thoughts
   - Is this a thought that helps us conduct ourselves effectively within the situation when we cling to it?
   - If we let the thought take the lead, will it lead us towards a full, meaningful life or just leave us stuck?
3. Notice when we cling on to a thought and when we succeed in parting from it.

> *I am not my thoughts*

IDENTIFYING CLINGING

In order to be able to conduct the process of separating from our thoughts, it is important to identify the clinging itself, what fields of life it occurs in, and how it manifests itself in six key issues: rules, reasons, judgment, past, future, and self.

Rules

What strict rules tell us how we should feel before we take certain action? Try distinguishing key words that are repetitively recurring like must, need, essential, right, wrong, don't, can't, I feel this way, I can't do this, if I do X you'll do Y, etc.

These words signify rigidity and affixation. They create suffering when adhered to. "I have to eat breakfast." "If I had a large meal I will have to work out." "I'm not allowed to have any pizza." "If I have a piece of cake I'll surely eat the whole thing." "I have to cut down on carbs."

Reasons

What reasons do we present to prove that change is simply impossible? "There is no way I'll manage to give up my wish to be thin." "I'm so tired of trying to lose weight, I don't have the energy for another process." "I'm not emotionally available." Adhering to these thoughts creates rigidity which does not allow change.

Judgment

When we cling to thoughts like: "I'm fat." "I'm lazy." "I'm a bad person." Or "I'm so selfish," our lives become full of struggle and suffering. It is important to identify which judgmental beliefs we adhere to. "I have no willpower." "I'm a failure." "I can't stick with anything." It is important to recognize that this is type of self-judgment is useless.

The Past

To what extent do we cling to the past? Recreating past failures, disappointments, mistakes, losses, or missed opportunities and, alternately, reminiscing about the amazing things we experienced in the past. Thoughts like "I wish I was like I was when I was 20 again." "I should've kept the weight off back then." "I'll only be truly happy when I return to my old weight."

Future

To what extent do we adhere to the future? We fear what will happen, fantasize about a better life. We constantly get caught up in thoughts of what we have to do. "If I don't lose weight I'll be ill." "I have to lose weight if I want to be hired for a new job."

"Self"

To what description of our self do we adhere? For instance: "I am weak and worthless." "I don't need help." "I'm nothing without my job." "I can't stick with anything." And alternately, to what body image or diagnosis we cling to: "I'm fat." "I'm depressed."

Identifying the process of sticking to thoughts or situations is vital in order to begin separating from them. This separation is not a technique, but a process, and the purpose of the different techniques is to help learn and enable the process to take place.

TECHNIQUES AND METHODS TO HELP ACHIEVE COGNITIVE DEFUSION

EXERCISE: THREE MINUTES OF THOUGHTS

Over the course of three minutes try to write down all of the thoughts that pass through your mind. With the help of this exercise you will be able to discover the amount of your passing thoughts and their speed.

The thought identification process can be translated to

a sketch on paper or an audio recording. Don't write the thoughts down word for word. Write down only a word or two that will remind you of the essence of the thought. Note how many thoughts you can capture in three minutes. Even if you started thinking about the exercise, write down the thought that popped up about it. Try to be honest with yourselves. When you're done, please count the number of thoughts and multiply by twenty. This way you can gauge the amount of thoughts that go through your mind in one hour.

QUESTIONS YOU CAN ASK:

- Is the clinging to a certain thought helpful? Does it lead you to take effective actions which benefit your well-being?
- For example, does clinging to the thought that you must be thin in order to meet a romantic partner help you work towards the life you want to live?
- Is this thought familiar to you? Have you seen it before?
- What do you gain from clinging to the story your thought tells you?

For example- what do you gain from adhering to a thought that claims if you walk for an hour each day you will lose weight?

INTERVENTIONS WHICH ALLOW DISTANCING:

The following three exercises are based on the realization that the nature of thought is to come and go.

"Clouds"- Imagine you are sitting in a field and watching the clouds go by. Lay a thought on each cloud and let it move on and away.

"River"- Imagine you are sitting by a flowing river.

Watch the water moving down the channel. Note the leaves floating on the water. Place a thought on each leaf and let it flow away.

"Sea sand"- Imagine you are sitting on the beach. Write the thought in the sand, and watch the waves rolling up the beach wash that thought away.

NOTICE WHAT YOUR MIND IS TELLING YOU RIGHT AT THIS MOMENT

This is a simple exercise which helps distance thoughts without getting involved with them. It invites us to observe what the mind has to say in this moment in the most direct way.

NOTICE THE SHAPE OF THE THOUGHT

This exercise is about visualization. It helps us look at our thoughts from a distance and ask questions that will maintain it. Can you see the thought, imagine its shape? What does it look like? What is it similar to?

We can also focus on the voice and ask "What does the thought sound like?" "Is it your voice or someone else's?" "Is it a loud or a quiet voice?" "Is it a soft voice?" "What is the emotion you are able to hear in it?"

I HAVE A THOUGHT

The ability to separate the thought from the person is essential. You are not your thoughts. This friendly exercise has a number of stages:

- "I have a thought that says…"- complete with a negative self-judgment to form a short sentence- "I am X." For example: "I have a thought that says 'I'm- lazy, I lack willpower, I'm incorrigible.' "

- Now cling to this thought for 10 seconds. Let it fill all of you.
- Now repeat this thought a second time but add a few words at the beginning of it. For example:
- "I notice that I have a thought that says I'm an incorrigible fatty."
- Now add another stage. And say, "I notice I see this thought that says…" what happened? Did you notice that distancing occurred and you could actually observe the thought without it becoming part of you? If not, repeat this exercise again with a different thought.

LEMON, LEMON, LEMON

This exercise has three steps:
- Take a simple noun like lemon. Say it out loud twice. Note what thoughts, images, scents, flavors, and memories automatically appeared.
- Now repeat the word lemon again and again, louder and faster for 30 seconds, until it becomes a meaningless sound.
- Now repeat this exercise over and over using judgmental words you use when you are criticizing yourself like "fat," "lazy," or "loser."

COMPUTER SCREEN

This exercise is useful for those of us who have visual abilities.
- Cling to a judgmental thought for 10 seconds- for example, "I'm incorrigibly fat."
- Imagine a computer screen and visualize your thought is written on it in black and white.

- In your mind, play with the colors of the font your thought is written in.
- Next, play with the size and shape of the font. Imagine your thought is written in Italian, Spanish, Chinese, or another language.ers. .
- Finally, visualize your negative, judgmental thought as having black letters and try, only with your eyes, to make the words dance and move as if they were animated cartoon characters.

IMAGINING

There are many methods to seeing thoughts with our mind's eye. The ability to imagine them in different ways creates distance and separation.

- We can imagine the thoughts as passing cars, speeding by our house as we look out the window.
- We can imagine the thoughts as water flowing through a fountain.
- We can imagine the thoughts as leaves blowing in the wind.

HOW OLD IS THE THOUGHT?

Whenever you think a familiar and painful thought, ask yourself, ""How old is this thought?" Try to recall the first time it appeared. This will remind you that it is just a thought; it has appeared in the past and will probably keep coming and going from time to time as it has before.

HOW DOES THIS THOUGHT SERVE ME?

When a thought grasps you, ask yourself, "How does it serve me?" What does my mind want me to do? Whenever a thought seeps into you, notice if it's trying to protect you from a scary situation, to prevent you from doing something that may trigger anxiety. This way you will not let your mind fool you.

"THANK YOU MIND"

This is a simple and easy distancing technique. You thank your mind each time an unpleasant thought jumps into it. This is a simple way to remind yourselves that this is just a thought. "I am so fat"- Thank you mind
"I'm such a good for nothing"- Thank you mind
"I will always be made fun of"- Thank you mind
"I'm anxious and nervous"- Thank you mind

THE WHITE ROOM MEDITATION

Find a quiet place to practice in, so no one will interrupt you. Sit down and close your eyes. Imagine your mind is a white room with two doors. Your thoughts enter from one door and exit from the other. When each thought crosses the room, watch it indifferently and label it: "Depressing thought"…."Thought about my mother"…."Guilty thought"…and note when the thoughts linger. This happens when you start believing them. Afterward, write down what happened or what failed. This exercise allows you to practice the act of labeling thoughts as a simple and effective skill.

MIRROR MIRROR

The mirror has become a battlefield for many people

who have a hard time looking at their reflection and thinking "Look at yourself." "What's that fat stomach?" "You have to lose 2 kilos." "You have so many wrinkles." "What is with that butt?" along with countless other words of criticism and guilt.

To us, being angry at ourselves seems to be effective for self-change. We also believe that we deserve this hurtful treatment and thus replicate what society is doing to us. We somehow become our own harshest critics. This exercise has two purposes: To bring up all of the thoughts that accompany standing in front of the mirror and to let them be "just thoughts." As such, we can allow them to come and go without grasping onto them and without being governed by them.

Please stand in front of a full-length mirror. Note, without speaking, the emotions that arise in you. Try to continue standing in front of the mirror and being in tune with your emotions. Note the thoughts that appear while continuing to look at yourself in the mirror. Focus on the eyes gazing back at you. Be quiet. Observe. Focus on the experience of observing. Note your thoughts and let them go.

After a few minutes of silent observation ask, yourself what you saw in the mirror. Describe the external components. Shoes, sweater, jewelry. Describe them without judgment. Then raise your gaze up along the body and attach a judgmental thought to every part of it. While you say them, distance yourself from the thought by saying, "I have a thought that says..." like, "I have a thought that says my hips are wide and large." Write down these thoughts. At the end of the exercise, try to distinguish what you feel and what thoughts are going through your head.

When you've finished this part of the exercise, sit down and read aloud all of the thoughts that you have written down before you.

NOTICE HOW THE THOUGHTS SPEAK THE LIES OF THE DIET LANGUAGE

For instance, let's focus on the thought: "If I ate pizza I'll be fat." We have four options:

Thinking in the Diet Language and promising yourself that you won't eat anything today or that if you dare eat you'll cut down or go to the gym afterwards, doing anything to maintain caloric balance.

Argue with the thought and theorize about why it isn't true. For example: "Why I won't be fat if I ate this pizza."

Try to think up a different, less threatening thought that will create relief, even if momentarily, from the guilt and the fear. Like, "Well, I only had one slice."

All of these techniques require much emotional and cognitive effort. In some way or other they keep us increasingly preoccupied with eating. The fourth option is:

Don't argue with these thoughts, don't test their truth, only test to what extent you cling to them and ask yourself if clinging to them promotes your well-being. There is always the option of just letting the thought go. Try doing so.. It's true new thoughts will always come, but you can always choose to act in a similar way with them.

> *The ability to let go of these thoughts is the ability to observe them instead of being in them*

IF I AM NOT MY THOUGHTS, THEN WHO AM I?

"You don't understand anything," she huffed at me. "You and your fifty kilos.Have you ever been fat?" she ranted on. "You look at me, I am what every possible failure looks like. Always losing weight but always gaining it back. I have never worn jeans. I have never bought myself a slinky negligee. And sex?

Always in the dark. So they don't see, so they don't know. And you're so skinny. It's easy for you to tell me to let go of my thoughts, to see them from outside. This has been my reality for years."

"What's letting go of these thoughts?" she continued. "And what will happen to me if they disappear just like that? My head will suddenly be empty if I don't constantly think about what I ate, how much, and why? I don't hate myself. I'll probably be much fatter. I have lived all my life like this. Thinking and breathing diets, anxiety, guilt. Counting and weighing. This sets my mood, this is my calling card, so how can I just let these thoughts go? But they're right, aren't they? Bread is really fattening and pizza is forbidden? And a thin person really is better and more worthy, isn't he?" She started to cry.

"For years these have been my thoughts," she confessed. "For years I am convinced they are right. For years they have been telling me who I am and what I am...for years. And if I won't be thin, and if I have actually wasted years fighting my body for nothing? Do you really think I wasted my time for nothing? That nothing will come out of this? That I hate myself for no reason?"

I said nothing. I looked at her. At the pain in her eyes, at her sunken shoulders, at the helpless limpness she posed at this moment.

"And how do you let go?" she asked "How do you stop doing more of the thing you are so accustomed to? Thoughts...thoughts...an assortment of words, you said? That I am the one who gives them meaning, right?" I nodded, hypnotized. Enchanted by the way in which her associations built upon one another and seemed to be opening a door to another way of looking at things, giving her a detached sense of observation which allowed her some kind of choice.

She leaned back in the chair, relaxed her body, and said, "You know, I'm not even sure I want to be thin. If I'm skinny no one will see me. And maybe my face will suddenly be long and my beauty will disappear? I've never been thin. I've been chasing this weight for forty years but I've never experienced any real success. Maybe these thoughts that I have adopted and lived by have really locked me up in this narrow world that is not really who I am?

Do you believe I can live without these thoughts? Will I just have a bit of quiet in my mind? Maybe I'll suddenly be different? A little happier, a little freer, more real?"

I didn't really know what my place was in the therapy room. She had connected all the dots on her own. She was strong, present. "I think I'm starting to see," she said. "These thoughts are coming and going. There are so many of them. But they are suddenly like raindrops on the window. Sliding down, dissipating. And you can see the view behind them. And there are people out there, and cars driving by, trees, sky, and other people's lives. I suddenly want to experience them so badly."

I smiled.

THE OBSERVING SELF

"And plants are just plants, not thinkers.
I can say this makes me superior to them
Or I can say it makes me inferior.
But I say nothing. I say of the stone, "It's a stone".
I say of myself, "It's me".
And I say no more. What more is there to say?"[61]

The observing self involves observing the mind, and reaching a point of view from which we observe thoughts and emotions without getting caught up in them.

The purpose- to help the individual stop identifying himself with his thoughts about himself.

The method- continuous practice of mindfulness techniques.

When to use it- when there is a need to support acceptance. When we are afraid of getting hurt by our own experiences and attempts. Or when we are really "stuck" to our thoughts about ourselves or about reality and are devoid of choice.

This dimension is meant to focus the three dimensions mentioned so far. Acceptance, being in the here and now, and cognitive defusion on one important, main, and elusive element: the self. The psychological ability this process attempts to create is distinguishing between the "true" transcendental self (beyond consciousness), that is impossible to conceptualize or define its limits, and the verbal self, the one that is conceptualized by the mind.[62]

The different labels we put on ourselves ("Depressive," "Obsessive," "Idiot," "Lacking confidence," "Always ruining everything," "Devoted father," "Perfectionist," "A good friend"), whether they are traits, pathologies, or other descriptions, whether they are perceived as negative or positive, are impossible to prove or dispute and are always superficial and one-dimensional.

The "observing self" is the one who can watch and observe the thinking self and the physical self. They are changing, but the observing self does not change. It becomes a safe and secure place. A place from which we watch over what is happening in the body and the mind without getting hurt.

NOTICE YOU ARE NOTICING

Rene Descartes is famous for saying "I think, therefore I am", but who is this "I" who notices this thinking? Here's a little exercise.

Watch X

There is X and there is you watching X

If you can watch X you cannot be X

X is continuously changing. You, who notice X is changing, are not changing.

X= your breathing, your thoughts, your feelings, the sensations in your body, the rules you live by

The observation process tells us there is a point of view that is outside the "self." A point from which we can watch over that X. That point never changes. The individual can watch thoughts, feelings, the body, the world around him, and even himself watching them. This point is like the sky, covered in clouds. Although we can't see the sky through the clouds covering them, we know they are always there.

- The observing self is not a thought or emotion; it is a point of view from which we can watch thoughts and emotions.
- When the person feels, thinks, senses, does- that part of him is always there and is aware of it.
- Without the observing self there will be no sustainability of self-consciousness.

- Thoughts and images rapidly change. At times they are pleasant, at times they are painful, at times they are efficient, at times bothersome. But one thing that is certain is the knowledge that they always come, and always change.
- The individual is constantly changing, but the observing self does not.

THE QUALITIES OF THE "OBSERVING SELF":

- The observing self is not judged as good or bad. Right or wrong. Since all it does is observe.
- The observing self makes a person aware of his actions and their consequences.
- The observing self will never judge, since judgment is a thought and the observing self cannot think.
- The observing self watches thoughts but does not create them.
- The observing self cannot be hurt even if the body is ill or in pain. It will simply notice it.
- Not bad thoughts, not suffering, not difficult feelings- nothing can change the observing self that watches them- that self is unchanging, is always there from the moment you notice its existence till the moment you die. Even if we think we have forgotten its existence.
- The observing self is not a thing- it has no physical qualities. It cannot be measured. Only each of us can know of the existence of the observing self out of personal experience.
- You cannot improve the observing self in any way- that is why it is always perfect.

- If I am not my mind then who am I? I am the combination of the thinking, physical, and observing self.

The camera allows us to acquire the skill of the observing self. It allows us pure observation. The camera gives us perspective, gives up power. The ability to observe the mind is a fascinating ability which exposes every individual to the world of thoughts and feelings.

SEEING

Take a camera, remember to push the record button and observe. See the thoughts, emotions, physical sensations without getting involved with them, without judging, without drowning in them. Only watching them. Seeing the body with its wrinkle, with its rolls of fat, the downturned mouth. Seeing the thoughts of judgment and criticism about how you look. Seeing the commercials on TV and the icons of thinness and knowing that you am not like that, and you choose not to try to be like that. Seeing the fear of food, of the cake you ate, the ice cream or the delicious bread and butter. Seeing the anger nearing, accustomed to appear almost every second. Seeing the fear of letting go and not being part of the pursuit of a thin body. Seeing and seeing.

But who wants to see? It is easier to live on autopilot. With what we've grown so accustomed to. It's easier to go with the flow than lift our head up and think if we feel good in it or not. To see yourself walking, to see your heart beat, to see yourself eating, to see you are sad and to see how much you think you see but actually don't see at all.

Take a camera, remember to push the record button and observe. See the world fill with sounds, sights, voices, scents, and flavors. See your desire to put judgment and criticism on every thought, see your mind hustling and bustling, unable to stop. See the world suddenly take on a different meaning.

See with no purpose or goal, see because you have chosen to see.

See. Just see.

THE VALUES OF LIFE

"First
for a thousandth of a second
I knew for certain
the secret of life
even if forgetting descended on me
and I forgot the moment I remembered
and not a word remained
except the taste of knowledge"[63]

So far I have presented mindfulness and its four components: acceptance, cognitive defusion, being in the here and now, and the observing self. We will use them in light of values- which are a beacon for life.

Values are a sort of statement about what we want to do with life. What we want to support and how we want to act on a daily basis. Values lead to core principals which drive how we manage our lives.

The purpose- clarifying to ourselves what gives our life meaning or purpose. To use these values as the guidelines for our actions.

Our society is mission driven and goal oriented- things that can be measured. Because of this we tend to confuse values with goals. Values are the direction in which we want to move in life. Goals are just a tool on our way there.

It is important that we focus again for a moment on the confusion between goals and values. As noted earlier, goals, big as they may be, give concrete points which we can navigate to, but the value is the process that is never reached or done which is in actuality the real "goal."

It is a common mistake to think that values, like goals, are in the future. Everything a person does to serve the

164

value, including the choice itself and the awareness of making it, is moving towards the chosen value. Values, unlike goals, are about the present and are geared towards the present.

HOW DO WE CHOOSE VALUES?

Values are beyond right and wrong. They are also beyond good and bad. They are a way of completely expressing what is really valuable and important to us. On our way to define them we should distinguish what parts of life are really important to us. Here are ten main dimensions of meaning in life:

- Intimate relationships- the nature of the relationship, closeness, openness, love, and loyalty as it is important and meaningful to you.
- Parenting- what does being a mother or father mean to you? How to love, protect, teach, educate, listen?
- Education and study- values like truth, curiosity, development,
- Friends and social life- who's your best friend? How many good friends do you have? What do you like to do with your friends? How many new friends would you have made if fear, sadness, anger would not have blocked you? And what about love, security, loyalty?
- Health- what changes would you want to make in your life in terms of nutrition, physical activity, preventative checkups? What do you think about vitality, strength?
- Family of origin- how dear and important to you is your relationship with your parents and other relatives? How would you like this relationship to be? A relationship based on respect, admiration, love, acceptance?

- Spirituality- are you aware or connected to powers bigger and stronger than you? What about God, creation, nature, poetry?
- Community life and citizenship- what about giving back to the community you live in? Recreation and creation- how would you like your free time to look like? How do you reenergize yourself? What is important to you? Passion, joy, laughter, creativity?
- Work and career- a large part of the life we lead is in the workplace. What would you like to get from your job and what would you like to give in it? What is important to you in the workplace? Excellency, development, inventiveness, leadership?

There is great value in pausing every once in a while to examine the values leading our lives.

> *Values, unlike goals, are about the present and are geared towards the present*

Here are some exercises to help you discover your values:

THE MAGIC WAND

This is an exercise about what we really want. What is really important to us in the overall scope of things? What would we want to fight for? Imagine you are waving a magic wand which gives you approval from all the people in the world, and no matter what you do, they still love, respect, and admire you.

What would you do with your life?
How would you treat others?

Wave your wand and all of the painful thoughts, memories, and emotions are no longer there and have no influence on you.

What would you do with your life?

What would you start or stop? Do more or less?

How would you behave differently?

If we are watching you on video, what would you see and hear that would show us magic that has happened?

SPEECHES

Imagine your 18th birthday. Two or three people are giving a speech in your honor. They are talking about what you are to them.

WEALTH

You have inherited a fortune. What would you do with it? Who is there to appreciate the things you have purchased or done? How would you act towards all of the people coming to share your new life with you?

SO, VALUES ARE:

- In the here and now
- Need no justification
- Best to grasp onto lightly
- Chosen freely

WHAT DO WE NEED VALUES FOR?

Acknowledging our values gives meaning and direction to life. It allows us to examine the path we are walking on and evaluate it at any given time. If, for instance, one of the values you have recognized as important to you is intimacy, you can evaluate to what extent preoccupation with diets and weight loss attempts fits in with and reinforces this value. Is it possible that your battle against weight is hurting your intimate relationships?

Once the individual sees how he manages his life, his eating, and his interpersonal relationships and if they fit in with his values or misses them, he is given the choice.

SO SHE WON'T BE THIN

No. She can't count calories, weigh in, be angry, blame, account, balance, hate. She's tired of these hurtful words. She can't and it seems to her that she doesn't even want to. No diet...no...just no.

So she won't be thin.

She's not thin at all anyway. For 20 years she has been in this battle. For 20 years she has been losing it. She still remembers that when she went into the army she weighed 62. And now? The scale won't go lower than 80. So strange. She would sign off on that weight today.

So what if the commercials promise redemption and happiness as attainable only in a desired weight. So what if all of her friends don't stop mulling over what they ate, counting calories, and suffering diet-related agnst. She's not there anymore. And all of a sudden she doesn't even realize how she was there. How she wasted her days and time with this laconic, boring preoccupation. She chooses her words carefully. A bit amazed at this flood of thoughts. A bit frightened for a moment. Is this her? Is this really her?

She's in front of the mirror. Her gaze slides down her body. Sees her round bottom, her stomach that has gone up and down and up again. No, she's not tall either, and her breasts are those of a woman past 50, no longer proudly perking up. A few wrinkles are around her eyes,creases are at the side of her mouth.

Her diet is not working, but what will happen if she goes off it? She won't have anything? No horizon? What kind of life is a life without goals? Without objectives? Without challenges? And what does a life with no diet look like? Empty?

Scary.

She sees the fear.

The automatic desire to grab on to something.

The desire for someone to take responsibility over her. To tell her where, what, when, and how. To force her into a program, to manage her, to choose for her. For her to be angry with, to complain to, to cry to, to feel guilty and unworthy. Because of whom she'll suffer and stop her life from moving on. To have who and what to blame. Something to hold her and for her to hold on to. That will keep her from living like she might want to live.

Scary.

She sees the fear.

Letting go of the language is a choice. Partly logical and partly intuitive. There is responsibility in choice. It brings with it ambiguousness and loss of control. It brings with it beginnings and surprises.

This is also scary.

This is what it's like without a diet. You're allowed to be hungry and ask why. You're also allowed to be full and know from what. You're allowed to experiment, to feel, to question, to make mistakes, to be confused, just as much as you're allowed to enjoy, take pleasure, discover.

No diet.

So she won't be thin.

So she won't!

MINDFUL EATING

"Eating mindfully is eating while acknowledging the eating and everything the body experiences when eating. Knowing the naked truth. Because why do we dress or not? Watch what we eat and how we eat or not? Not only because we are embarrassed of others but first and foremost because we are embarrassed of ourselves.[64]*"*

- Do you eat even when you're full?
- Do you continue to snack until you feel physical discomfort?
- Do you avoid certain foods?
- Do you find yourselves snacking on foods even if you don't particularly enjoy them, just because they are in front of you or you have already paid for them?

If you answered yes to these questions, you probably tend to eat mindless. But the language of Mindful Eating, unlike the Diet Language, deals less with what to eat, how much, and when, and focuses instead on the "how" of it all. It is not eating that is full of intimidation, rules, and laws, but free, which allows us to eat what we want. Eating that tells us that it's okay to eat, that eating is delicious and important and an integral part of our life.

Therefore, Mindful Eating is:
- Not a diet or an eating plan full of rules
- Not another way of controlling food
- Not a path that necessarily leads to weight loss
- About how you eat more than what you eat

Mindful Eating is eating that involves all of the senses in the eating process. When we ignore what we see, touch, experience, or feel, eating is lost and is no longer present.

As such, it rarely provides the very values for which it exists- like satiation, fullness, or pleasure. **Mindful Eating** is eating that is led by tuning in to the true needs of the individual in the here and now.

Mindful Eating is flexible and varied eating which is affected by various aspects including health, cost, social situation, emotional state, comfort, allergy, environmental influence, taste, quality of food, vegetarianism, or carnivorism, the type of food, location, time. Mindful Eating is at its best when we understand that we cannot take into consideration all of these factors at once.

The key to Mindful Eating lies in the understanding that it is a combination of various factors which can exist without us feeling fear or shame.

Mindful Eating is based on the assumption that the body needs variety. Eating will be examined not in regard to food but always in regard to the feeling it awakes in the body.

Mindful Eating allows us to be present in the here and now when we eat. It is judgment-free awareness to the entire eating process, from start to finish.

Mindful Eating is like discovering magic. When we introduce mindfulness into the eating process, it becomes surprising, rich, satiating, and pleasurable.

MOST EATING LACKS MINDFULNESS AND ATTENTION

A study held among 29 female students checked if concentrating while eating enhances the memory of the meal and reduces food consumption later. The study included three groups: the treatment group- to whom a three minute long sound byte was played during the meal which included mindfulness techniques like an instruction to focus on the appearance, the scent, the taste, the texture, the aftertaste, and the source of the food served.

In addition, the participants were asked to concentrate on the act of chewing and swallowing. An additional group was asked to read an article about food while the control group was given no instruction or task. The three groups consumed the same meal, which included a sandwich and French fries and was allotted ten minutes to eat. The study's results found that the participants in the treatment group remembered their lunch more vividly in comparison to the two other groups. They also ranked themselves as less hungry two hours later. Later on, when they were utilizing the option of consuming three types of cookies, there was a complete correlation between the amount of cookies consumed and the vividness of the memory of lunch.

We often crave ice cream, grilled cheese sandwiches, or pizza, which are perceived as forbidden when dieting. A dissonance is created. On one hand is the craving and on the other is the prohibition. If we eat we transgress from the rules. If we don't eat we transgress from ourselves. From this moment the binge is just a matter of time. Because in order to eat the individual must "disappear" in order for him to not witness the "sin" he can't contain. This situation causes him to enter a cognitive dissociation which enables eating. This type of eating is devoid of pleasure, attention, and satisfaction, and is laced with guilt.

A study held among 554 students examined if mindfulness attributes health in terms of physical activity, quality of sleep, stress, and binge eating. The rate of eating binges among students is high. About 40% of male students and 20% of female students have reported binge eating. The findings pointed to a significant negative link between mindfulness and the frequency and severity of the binges, quality of sleep, and stress levels. A positive link was also found between mindfulness and engaging in and enjoying physical activity.

A study held among 26 women, whose average age was 48.5 and average weight was 94.6 kilos showed that practicing developing mindful, aware, and judgment free eating, developing awareness of physical sensations like hunger, satiation, desire, and stress, developing awareness of thoughts and emotions related to food, acceptance and lack of judgment towards thoughts, emotions and sensations and physical activity, leads to significant improvement. Improvement that is manifested in the frequency of emotional eating, a decrease in the desire for food and dichotomistic thinking and a decline in eating that stems from external factors and not a physical need.

Mindful, intuitive eating decreases the loss of control over eating and binge eating

---

IN ORDER TO REACH MINDFUL EATING WE MUST RECOGNIZE AND COMBINE:

- Feelings experienced before, during, and after we eat
- Thoughts that manage our eating
- Sensations in the body
- The eating process itself
- Self-perception
- The overt and covert, internal and external system of rules regarding food and body

WHY IS IT SO DIFFICULT TO DEVELOP MINDFUL EATING?

Our mind is programmed to notice patterns, so events deviating from the pattern are not absorbed as easily as predictable events are absorbed. In the human mind, expectations and goals are seamlessly woven into the basic processes of perception and they are not easy to undo. Expectations are based on previous experiences and the perception is based on these expectations. Experience and expectations help us organize what we see.

Christopher Chabris and Daniel Simmons, the authors of the book *The Invisible Gorilla*[65], talk about a certain kind of blindness that is not caused by a visual impairment. They are talking about cognitive blindness- not noticing unexpected figures that appear right where we're looking because our attention is turned elsewhere. The famous *Invisible Gorilla* experiment includes a video showing two groups of people tossing a ball back and forth. One of the teams is wearing white shirts, and the other black shirts. The participants were asked to quietly count the passes only between the players in the white shirts. While they were watching, a student dressed as a gorilla casually walked into the circle of people playing, stopped among them, turned to the camera, pounded on her chest, and left. Her appearance lasted nine seconds. Once the video was over, the participants were immediately asked to report how many passes they counted. The task of counting was meant to occupy the participants with an activity that demands attention, in order to see if the test subjects would notice the gorilla's surprising entrance. Most of them missed it.

The researchers claimed we have difficulty noticing things that are unexpected. The amount of information we screen is vast. Most of us suffer from "blindness to change," which is linked to our inability to compare what we see to what we remember seeing. A disconnect is created between what we think about the act of remembering and what actually is.

Our memory does not store everything we perceive, it takes what we saw or heard and links it to what we already know. Simmons and Chabris talk about six illusions of attention: the illusion of attention, memory, confidence, knowledge, cause, and potential. All of these regard the distorted beliefs the individual has about his mind, to which he clings. Understanding this may explain in part the difficulty in developing Mindful Eating. Eating that becomes difficult when met with the complexity of the human mind and its very real difficulty to be present in the here and now.

The principle of pleasure, as defined by Freud, also weighs on our ability to "just be." In any given moment we are trying to seize the moment of pleasure and prevent the moment of pain. Because of this it is nearly impossible to feel satisfied. Take a minute to try and recreate the last 24 hours. In what moments were you really in the moment, valuing it, experiencing it to its fullest?

EXERCISE- PAUSING THOUGHTS

Close your eyes, and please try for one minute to stop the flow of thoughts. Try to see if you can remember words that have been created in your mind. What happened?

Most people find that it's difficult for them to stop thinking. Please write down some of the thoughts that have come in. If you pay attention to the thoughts, you will find that most of them are about the past or the future and combine thoughts and expectations with the goal of increasing pleasure and decreasing pain.

HOW DO WE LEARN TO DEVELOP MINDFUL EATING?

"The mind, that was used for so long to be turned outside, is not easily turned inside. It is difficult to limit a cow that is used to grazing in other fields to its own pen. Even if her owner tempts her with delicious grass and excellent feed, it refuses at first, then eats a little bit, but her innate tendency to roam overcomes her and she fails. When her owner tempts her over and over again, she slowly becomes

accustomed to the pen. Finally, if she's released, she will not roam.
The human mind is the same.[66]

The perception that the individual can trust his internal signals of eating without external intervention was first documented in 1928 by Clara Davis, a child development researcher, who found that babies demonstrate an innate ability to control their food consumption on the caloric and nutritional level. She found that eating habits are individual. Leann Birch also showed in her studies that newborn babies know to manage their food consumption independently. She showed that external intervention in children's eating disrupts this innate ability. Indeed, a newborn baby acts out of full attention to his natural codes: he cries when he's hungry and sleeps when he's full. These codes are disrupted throughout life, when attention and confidence gradually make way for external rules and codes: parents, social pressure, diets, the pursuit of thinness, medicalization of eating and environmental strictures. All of these disrupt and halt the natural hunger and satiation mechanism.

Acquiring ownership over hunger is an individual process that changes from one person to another. You cannot identify true hunger and satiation in the attempt to lose weight. As long as weight loss is what governs the body, the individual will continue eating according to what the scale shows him and try to eat as little as possible.

The beginning of the process of becoming aware of your eating and developing attention to hunger and satiation is first and foremost to accept it as it is. Without wanting to change it. This process of acceptance is done using six dimensions. Acceptance, observation, expansion, allowance, normalization, and self-compassion.

- **Acceptance**

Acceptance is an essential condition on the path to developing Mindful Eating. Acceptance does not signal concession, it enables the ability to let go of ineffective perceptions, beliefs, and rules, in order to open the door and allow significant change to take place. It enables us to be able to see eating as it is, to know the language governing it and to see the way in which we eat because of it. It is eating that provides health, fullness, and pleasure.

There is something scary and complex about this process, but it is also fascinating.

- o Scary, as a result of the discovery. Because we acknowledge the language that governs us and our eating.
- o Complex, because of the combination between the four dimensions of mindfulness- acceptance, being in the here and now, witnessing the mind, and cognitive defusion.
- o Fascinating, as a result of the path.

- **Observation**

Observing thoughts, emotions, and sensations that appear before, during, and after eating. The most useful tool for developing this skill is the journal. Its purpose is not to judge or criticize and not to evaluate, analyze, or count calories. It is just a way which allows us to meet eating, to make it as present as possible and to not run away from it as most people do.

- **Expansion**

A process which gives a place to eating and the thoughts and feelings that accompany it while letting go of the struggle against it and the need to tune it or control it. This is the ability of allowing ourselves to be wholly present while eating.

- **Allowance**

Acceptance does not mean concession and it also doesn't mean that you have to love what you see or want it. But it does mean allowing it to be as it is. There is no need to run away, hide, to be afraid or ashamed. The goal is not to change eating. The goal is to be able to allow it to exist, be realized, and just be present as it is. Because of this it might change, but it might not.

- **Normalization**

Acceptance enables normalization. Normalization enables acceptance. As long as eating is perceived as a sin and a weakness, the person eating is perceived as guilty and weak. Accepting eating as it is, accepting the body as it is, will make the struggle against them redundant. It will make them legitimate, allowed and thus, normal, worthy.

- **Self-compassion**

Self-compassion is the ability to be caring and look after yourself. It reduces the use of the inner critic and opens up the option for us to be more at ease with ourselves, which deepens the acceptance process.

The use of these dimensions does not have to occur in a particular order or in dictated and set amounts. It can change according to your needs. The use of them might change eating but it might not. But as previously stated, that is okay, because the purpose is not to change eating or decrease food consumption, but to accept it. To allow it to be as it is, without struggle. When we don't invest so much effort, time, and energy in trying to control eating, we can invest our energy in listening to it, being in it, making the most of it and giving the body what it deserves.

The desire to lose weight does not allow us to learn the natural codes of hunger and satiation

The process of identifying hunger and satiation is divided into four stages:

STAGE A- IDENTIFYING HUNGER

Hunger is meant to serve, first and foremost, as an alarm system. The initial signs of hunger serve as a signal system and they are not strong. When ignored, they will turn off for a little while, since the body knows that the need for food is not urgent. With time the signals get stronger and they don't calm down until you actually eat.

Some people can ignore them almost completely (dissociation). In this situation they will not feel true hunger even when the body really is hungry. But once they start eating and their attention will be focused on hunger and its satiation, it will lead to loss of internal eating control and make it difficult for them to stop eating (like after a fast or when going off a diet).

Every healthy person gets hunger signals on a daily basis, even if he's overweight. But when he ignores them on a regular basis they become useless to the extent of turning off. People learn to temporarily ignore these signals and they will later have difficulty recreating them.

Identifying hunger is an individual process that differs from one person to the other. It requires focus on eating and developing mindfulness to it with no criticism or guilt in the here and now.

When we identify we're hungry we are supposed to feel it in our body. These physical sensations are followed by thoughts like, "How do I know I'm hungry?" "Am I allowed to eat?" "When did I last eat?" "What should I eat so I don't gain weight?" "Maybe I'll try to wait a little bit more?" "Maybe I'll have something small and only allow myself a full meal for dinner?" Most of us find it difficult to stop and ask very practical questions about the hunger itself, like: "Is this physical hunger?" "How hungry am I?" "What do I want to eat right now that will make me feel comfortable physically?" "What will satiate me?"

Most thoughts wander to external discourse, based on allowed and forbidden, need and don't need, external rules that will allegedly lead us to control over our eating. This discourse misses our attention to our bodies, misses its true needs. This type of eating does not satisfy us in most cases and leaves us feeling lacking and deprived. These feelings can lead us to binge eating and loss of control over our eating habits in general. That is why in this stage we will try to identify hunger while focusing on the experience in the moment. We'll ask "Am I even hungry?" "If so, what kind of hunger is this, emotional or physical?"

STAGE B- IDENTIFYING THE DEGREE OF HUNGER

Identifying the degree of hunger is done using the hunger and satiation scale. The scale is based on the assumption that everyone is born with natural codes of hunger and satiation, they instruct us when to start eating and when to finish. The hunger and satiation scale moves on a numeric grade from zero to ten.

It is recommended to start eating when you are not hungry (between stage three and stage four) and finish eating when you're not too full (between stage six and stage seven).

THE HUNGER AND SATIATION SCALE

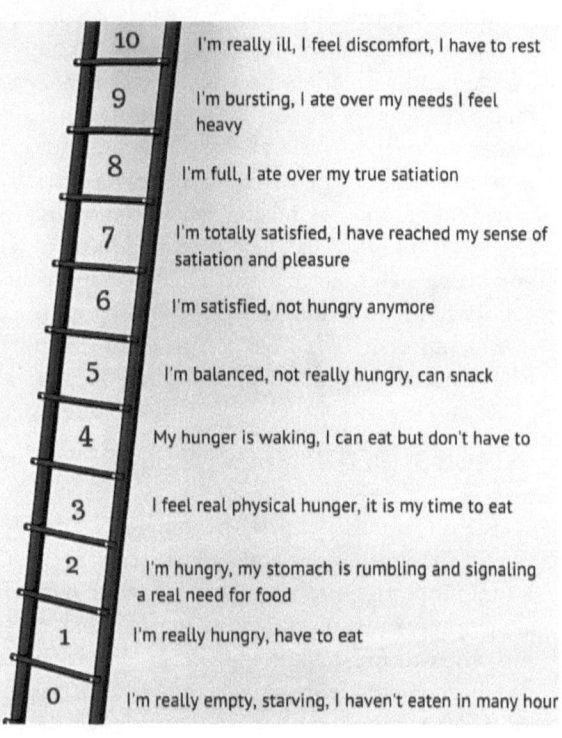

10	I'm really ill, I feel discomfort, I have to rest
9	I'm bursting, I ate over my needs I feel heavy
8	I'm full, I ate over my true satiation
7	I'm totally satisfied, I have reached my sense of satiation and pleasure
6	I'm satisfied, not hungry anymore
5	I'm balanced, not really hungry, can snack
4	My hunger is waking, I can eat but don't have to
3	I feel real physical hunger, it is my time to eat
2	I'm hungry, my stomach is rumbling and signaling a real need for food
1	I'm really hungry, have to eat
0	I'm really empty, starving, I haven't eaten in many hour

STAGE C- WHY ARE WE HUNGRY?

At this stage we distinguish what would really satiate our hunger. We can ask the following questions:

- What food are we hungry for?
- Would my choices be different if food didn't affect weight or health?
- What considerations, beliefs, myths, needs, guide us in choosing the food?
- Do we want something salty, sour, sweet, or spicy?
- Do we need hot or cold food?
- Do we want crunchy or soft food?
- Do we need proteins or carbohydrates?

If we listen to our body, we discover that it knows how to balance itself and that in states of physical hunger only real food will quiet it. The precise choice of food that we are hungry for will help us reach the right satiation and be comfortable with it.

STAGE D- IDENTIFYING SATIATION

Working with the hunger and satiation scale teaches us that it is easier to recognize when to start eating, but more difficult to recognize when to finish.

The real point of satiation is a sensation of satisfaction and comfort with a touch of pleasure and no traces of hunger. This is a private sensation which is located in the solar plexus, near the pyloris- where the esophagus enters the stomach. Eating with observation and real attention to the food, the taste, the texture and the sensations food arouses helps identify the point of satiation. Maimonides also addressed this issue at the time, and according to him we should eat up to a quarter of the stomach's fullness. To reach that point where within 20 minutes you feel a pleasant satiation in your body. As long as you eat exactly what you're hungry for, the satiation becomes more precise and more satisfying.

Real satiation is a combination of fullness and pleasure

EXERCISE- MINDFUL EATING

The next exercise requires concentration, courage, and to the process which is not for granted. In order to enable Mindful Eating we must see the barring thoughts that threaten us in the Diet Language - and let them go. I invite you to ask yourselves "What are those scary thoughts saying?" "To what extent does grasping on to them promote beneficial eating?" and then choose whether to hold on to them or let them go. Whether to live our life by them or not. Once we make room for mindfulness (despite the fears) it can help us, contain, be compassionate. It can allow dietetic thoughts to come and go without fighting them and without wanting to change them. It will help us see our eating not in their light. From the right view will come the right action.

MINDFULNESS WITH A PIECE OF CHOCOLATE

Please take two chocolate cubes (pieces). Place them beside you. Sit comfortably on a chair or armchair and try to focus on the exercise. Take one cube and hold in it your hand. Look at it carefully, notice its texture and color. Note the thoughts and feelings that arise in you as you hold it..

Now, use your thumb and forefinger to examine the texture of the chocolate (you can also close your eyes in order to concentrate even more). Examine the lumpiness in the chocolate. Is it soft or hard, smooth or rough? Now, slowly raise it to your nose. Inhale and try to recognize its aroma. Try to recognize the emotions accompanying the scent. Are they pleasant, are they unpleasant, or are they neutral?

Inhale several times, smell the chocolate. Now bring the chocolate to your lips and let your tongue reach it. Let the chocolate rest between your tongue and your upper lip for a moment. Note the way your mouth reacts. Note every sensation that arises. Keep holding the chocolate like this for a minute or two. Now let your tongue explore it. Note how the chocolate changes in your mouth. Once you notice that you have explored the chocolate enough with your tongue, gently place it between your jaws. Hold the chocolate between your teeth and note the sensation. Note the urge to bite the chocolate and maybe even save it. Now let your teeth close just once. Note what happens. Note the experience of the taste, the urge, and the feelings that arise. Continue to explore the chocolate as it is chewed by your teeth.

After the chocolate has disintegrated in your mouth, go on chewing and note the change in the feelings and urges that arise. Note the swallowing reflex and the changing sensation. Follow the chocolate as it slides down your esophagus into the stomach, until it disappears.

Now take the second chocolate cube and note the thoughts that run around. Note what the mind has to tell you and what the sensations are in your body, in your mouth. Do you really want that cube? Maybe you choose to eat it from different reasons- like simply the fact that the chocolate is here and it's free?

If you found that you want the second cube, eat it in a similar fashion, with mindfulness and pleasure.

When you are done with the exercise, ask yourself:

- What thoughts and feelings did you have before, during, and after the exercise?

185

- What did your body signal to you before, during, and after the exercise?
- Did you eat both cubes of chocolate?
- Did you eat because you wanted it or because it was there?
- What was the taste and pleasure like in the second cube as opposed to the first?

The inner permission to eat allows us the satiation and the pleasure from it

---

EATING AS LOVEMAKING

Eating, in many senses, is like lovemaking. Entwined in it is an existential need to survive, pleasure, flourish. As well as desire and lust. Also innate to it is a constant dissonance between allowed and forbidden, overt and covert, legitimate and illegitimate.

We crave it, need it, run from it, hide from it, avoid it, attack it. We have a hard time acknowledging its uncompromising existence in our lives and more so to give it inner license.

She laid the sandwich on the plate before her. Looked at it. A sandwich full of good stuff. Goat's cheese, grilled peppers, tomato spread, lettuce. Wrapped in opaque parchment paper, cut in half.

She's a bit embarrassed. Eating in front of me? Without me eating as well? It's like standing naked in front of the mirror. How can she? It is so intimate. So personal, so charged. So illegitimate.

I placed a napkin by her side and made her a cup of tea. This will make the eating ritual more luxurious, more complete, and I invited her to look inside her body. What does she feel inside it? How hungry is she? To what extent did she really choose what she most wants to eat right now?

I explained that eating is divided into three parts, like lovemaking. It includes foreplay, the experience of the intercourse itself, and the orgasm. Every stage and its place. It can be a sort of one night stand which provides some sort of pleasure, but it can also be a full ceremony, every single stage of which is pure pleasure. They are both legitimate, and you have a choice in each one of them. Because what is the point of eating if it did not leave any impression of fullness and pleasure?

And she looked at me and at the sandwich across from her. Her eyes frosting over as she stared. "You want me to enjoy this sandwich?" she asked "How can I?I'm not allowed to eat bread, and surely not goat's cheese, which is full of calories." I replied, "But this is what you chose to eat, this is what you most wanted, right?"

"Right," she said, "the fact that I wanted it doesn't mean I can allow myself to enjoy it. It was always on the forbidden list, or at least the restricted one." I smiled at her. I saw the stress in her eyes, I tried to relax her, to let her unravel. "Part of the process is this inner license to eat everything, to enjoy everything. Without it, eating will forever remain in the Diet Language - full of guilt.

But like in sex, it is difficult to enjoy it if you do not allow it to exist if you are not really present in the experience, if you don't feel worthy of this pleasure, if you don't choose it. Sex is complete pleasure, and so is eating. This pleasure is what makes food satiating. Without it we will always stay hungry. Unsatisfied."

"And back to the foreplay," I went on. "It requires observation with all of your senses of the food we intend to eat...observing the texture, the scent.You can also feel it...a sort of process of acquainting ourselves with this food that we have always eaten automatically."

She opened her eyes wide and said, "I have never noticed food. I sometimes eat quickly while hiding, even from myself. Terrified of it and of the meaning it creates for me."

I looked at her, listening to her words...I saw the anxiety and the confusion, and said, "In the next stage, when the food is in your mouth I invite you to close your eyes and maximize the experience. Feel the chewing, the texture of the food, the types of food mixing in it. Don't rush to swallow. Let the food be there until you have experienced it to its fullest and only then allow it to slide down your esophagus and into your stomach. One bite followed by another bite. Slowly your stomach is filling and you can feel the experience of emptiness fading away.

Like an overturned hourglass the food slides down until the sensation of fullness will signal to you 'enough!' Remember that we are dealing with lovemaking. The love of eating, self-love."

"You really think I can stop eating when I'm full? What if I haven't finished my sandwich and my stomach will signal that it's full? What then? Do you really think I can pass on a part of it?" she said. I smiled. I understood where she was coming from. The anxiety, the panic...this new experience.

"And how will I know that I'm really full?" she asked. "You will discover the secret of this magic yourself," I continued. "There is fullness and satisfaction combined. That is the orgasm that you only know the magic of once you experience it. Everyone in his own way. The magic of eating is like the magic of love."

WHAT IF IT'S EMOTIONAL HUNGER?

"Feeling quiet
Feeling sounds
Feeling the rain
Feeling inside
Feeling the ground
Feeling to fly
What does it matter, just to feel again
Feeling pain
Feeling touch
Feeling the heart wrapped in love
Feeling colors
Feeling important
What does it matter, just to feel again." *

THE NATURE OF EMOTIONS

Emotions are signals found in our body which tell us what is happening. They developed with a special purpose, mainly to encourage the person to take actions that will help him survive, to keep him safe. Negative emotions are a sign that something wrong or scary is happening, which pushes the person to cope. In many senses, emotions are like a news service which gives constant updates about what is happening and how we are experiencing it. For instance, anxiety will urge us to avoid dangerous situations. Sadness will encourage us to slow down, retreat, and seek quiet in order to process loss or rebuild our strength after we fail. Shame will point to a demand to hide or stop something, which could end in resentment.

The initial reaction to what is happening is called a primary emotion. These are strong emotions that emerge quickly, before thoughts manage to come in. In response

---

* Arkadi Duchin, from the album "To Feel"

to the primary emotion there is also secondary emotion. In other words, it is an emotion about an emotion. For example, Michal yelled at her sister, who annoyed her and made her feel angry. The anger welled up in her immediately, but later she felt guilty about it. Anger was the primary emotion while guilt was the secondary emotion. You can feel endless secondary emotions in response to one primary emotion. It is also possible that the array of secondary emotions will cause greater pain and stress than the primary one. It is important then to try and diagnose what the primary emotion that set off the emotional escalation was so we will be able to cope with it before it develops and becomes a complex system of emotions.. We will touch on this later on.

HOW DO EMOTIONS WORK?

Emotions are chemical and electric signals in the body which signal to the person about what is happening. They have a role, and they're useful. They are very efficient as survival tools (fight or flight), they help change direction when we're facing a problem or new circumstances, remember people and situations, handling situations in everyday life, communicating with others, preventing pain and seeking after pleasure and joy. Emotions, no matter how powerful and confusing, accompany the individual throughout his whole life. They develop like waves. Rise up, peak, and recede. Their duration is limited.

When a person is in a whirlwind of emotions and it seems to him that this will last forever, he must remember that this is an illusion, caused by the power of emotions and sometimes by the need to push them away and be resilient against them. We experience countless different emotions every day.

You cannot control emotions. They are like thoughts. They come and go. Struggling with them, wanting to avoid them or needing to control them can intensify them and hurt us.

An emotional response is more than a mood or a feeling. It has four components:
- Effect
- Emotionally driven thoughts
- Physical sensations
- Emotionally driven behavior

Effect- The subjective experience of the emotions themselves as part of the changes in the body.

Emotion is a state of increase in the emotional and physical tone as a reaction to internal or external events. This reaction continues as long as the event continues to touch us. The effect is manifested in changes in facial features, posture, movement, speech, physical changes, pallor, or blushing.

The effect is what we call sadness, fear, anger, and anxiety. The mood is a given emotional state at a particular time which tints the way in which a person lives his internal and external world. The effect motivates certain action like attack or retreat. Negative emotions create a sense of discomfort, that things are not okay and we must fix them. This part of the effect is meant to grab our attention, so we acknowledge the fact that there is an unbalanced situation which requires action.

Emotionally driven thoughts- Thoughts about the situation we are in or about the emotions themselves. Thoughts that stem from an emotional reaction tend to divide into two groups: predictive thoughts and judging thoughts.

The predictive thoughts try to go into the future and understand what dangers it holds.They predict "What if...." While judging thoughts are about "What have I done? What's my fault?" When they are turned to yourself they will mostly cause sadness and depression.When turned to others they will cause anger. Emotionally driven thoughts can bring to life new additional emotions or intensify and provoke the initial ones.

Physical sensations- Every emotion has a physical element. We feel emotions in our body. Anxiety increases heartbeat, accelerates breathing, and it can cause perspiration, shaking, and tensing in the muscles. The feeling of depression includes heaviness, dullness, and exhaustion. Anger will create sensations of heat and tension in the arms and legs. Shame will lead to sensations of weakness, heat waves, and paralysis. The physical sensations that accompany each emotion can contribute to the feedback cycle and intensify the emotion.

Emotionally driven behavior- The urge to act always accompanies emotions. Anxiety, for instance, causes us to want to avoid things. Anger can cause aggression. Shame and guilt can lead to wanting to hide. There is something survivalist in these automatic actions but they can also lead us to an emotional complication which will cause us suffering.

HOW DOES AN EMOTIONAL PROBLEM ARISE?[67]

The creation of emotional problems is often blamed on stress, trauma, hormonal state, interpersonal conflicts, genetics and more....but another dimension must be added to these and that is the way in which we tend to cope with emotions. Every one of us has developed their own strategies in order to deal with the complexity of life.Some strategies work and some don't. Some create problems themselves. There are seven strategies which are usually used in situations of stress and emotional discomfort. Avoiding the experience, negative rumination, utilizing an emotional mask, focusing on a short-term solution, repeating a familiar reaction, hostility and hate, or negative assessment.

- Avoiding an experience- is avoiding painful thoughts and emotions. This is a coping mechanism which on many occasions is a double edged sword. Not only does it not suppress painful emotions, it increases them. Eating as a way to avoid feelings has long become routine for us.

- Rumination- regards the thoughts and behaviors that focus the individual on the symptom, its ramifications and its causes. There is no focus on solving the problems, but on the need to fear them. This is not thinking about how to get out or how to fix it next time. Rumination keeps the focus on what is bothering us, which intensifies bad feelings, anger, the anxiety and the hopelessness. An endless "mulling over" of "Why did I eat that?" "I look awful." "I'm so bad." Or "I'll always stay fat."

- Emotional mask (camouflage) - is the way to ensure that "No one will see my pain." Use of this strategy stems from the fear that others will see your emotions, judge them or criticize them and think that you are weak, stupid, crazy…the mask covers the harsh emotions that are raging inside you but must, allegedly, be hidden. And so the real self is hidden but is also left helpless. For instance, obesity can be an emotional mask; it can also be a disguise or create a sense of power and strength.

- Focusing on the short term- The thought behind this strategy is: "Why do it right when I can do it now?" When people experience emotional situations that they find difficult to be in, they search for instant relief. They want to immediately dim the emotion, to mask it or dull it down, and they will do anything that will allow them to put a wall up between them and their feelings. In most cases the relief is momentary. And in its next reincarnation the emotion will be more powerful and more painful. Food, for instance, is an efficient and instant comforter that serves wonderfully in the short-term, but is harmful in the long-term.

- Constant reaction- Recurring use of a certain response even if it isn't actually effective in a manner which creates rigidity and narrow mindedness. For instance, using food –or, alternately, dieting- to avoid feelings.

- Hostility, hate, aggression- These are efficient techniques to mask hiding, stress, anxiety, guilt, shame, or any sensation that hints that we have acted incorrectly. Anger, for instance, is a way to cover up a lot of pain in such a way that it keeps it far from our consciousness. This strategy is often efficient in the short term, but in the long term the angrier you are, the more you become a "grouch."

- Negative assessment- This is a way of "preparing" for failure or disappointment that may come. Focusing attention on the negative may seem efficient and something that protects us from pain. But like the other strategies, the use of it may be calming in the short-term, but becomes harmful in the long-term.

AVOIDING EMOTIONS[68]

Five types of avoidance exist:

- **Avoidance of situations**- Avoidance that allegedly protects us from meeting with people, places, objects, and activities that may arouse painful and uncomfortable emotions. A fat person, for instance, avoids going to the beach, shopping for clothes, eating delicious food, introducing himself to people. Some will avoid eye contact, meeting with strangers, meeting certain animals, family members, and so on.

- **Cognitive avoidance**- This avoidance takes place in the mind. We avoid stressful thoughts or memories by oppressing and repressing them. For instance, we tend to say to ourselves "Don't think about this; just don't go in that direction." Or we tend to push away unwanted images. This avoidance sometimes takes the shape of worrying too much. We can hold on to worrying about the future and living in its shadow while constantly imagining possible "what if…" scenarios while hoping that constant preparedness will prevent bad things from occurring in the future. Additional cognitive avoidance is replacing stressful thoughts or memories with other mental content. We can fill our mind with fantasies, dreams, or repetitive mental rituals like saying prayers for good luck again and again during the day.

- **Protective avoidance**- This avoidance describes the attempt to prevent dangers and risks with protective behavior, like checking locks, turning off lights, the gas switch, and so on. Or by carrying certain objects that give us a sense of protection like a cellphone we could use to call for help, talismans that have symbolic value or even anti-anxiety medication. Protective avoidance can also be compulsive cleaning, repetitive hand washing or perfectionism, for example. Dieting can also go on this list due to its strict nature and the way it makes many foods forbidden.

- **Somatic avoidance**- Through sensations like heat, lack of air or faintness we avoid feeling threatening feelings like sexual arousal or excitement before an event.
- **Avoidance as a substitute-** Replacing or impressing uncomfortable sensations with other emotions. Replacing anxiety with another strong emotion that is easier to handle, like anger. Other popular diversion tactics are binge eating, alcohol and drugs which allegedly dim or replace painful emotions. Gambling, dangerous extreme behaviors, video games...all provide an alternative means of avoidance.

All five avoidances have similar results. Although they provide pleasant relief in the short-term, in the long-term they create pain and suffering.

> *Emotions are like waves- they come and go. No matter what we feel and how strong and painful the emotion will be, it will pass*

EMOTIONAL EATING

Emotional eating is a type of avoidance. It is a way of feeling or not feeling the emotions we are scared to make room for. This is a behavior that is legitimate if only because it represents a deep natural need. But in the diet world it has been labeled a problem because it is disruptive to calorie counting, the weight loss process, and so on.

But we cannot prevent the arrival of emotions and our attempts to avoid feeling them usually don't work, they only increase the pain and the suffering, so using eating as a method of avoidance or distraction is doubtful. If so, it seems that the battle against emotions and the battle against emotional eating is a redundant one, because they are one and the same.

> *Labeling eating as emotional eating deprives it of its legitimacy and causes loss of control and binge eating*

NIGHTTIME EATING

She is single. 40 years old. Her name is Ronit. Her blond hair flows over her shoulders.

I have been accompanying her for years in her battle against her weight. Years during which every night she has been curling up with her cup of tea and her sweets. A fixed ritual. She sets the plate on the cushion at her side, and on it she carefully places the slice of cake - layers of chocolate with hints of cheese - and the paper napkin and the glass mug full of herbal tea. She is tired. Her day was packed with work and interest. She lightly taps at the remote and flips through the channels. Staring. For a moment her gaze pauses on this show or the other, but she continues to channel surf,uninterested. The tea is getting cold. She takes a bite of the cake, gently collects the crumbs from the corners of her mouth, making sure not to sully the cushion. She sips her tea. Pleasant warmth spreads through her body, which slowly relaxes as it gives in to the pleasure. Another bite...The news anchor talks about a shooting near Gaza, she's not really paying attention. The chocolate fills her with tranquility.

Her eyelids are heavy and she sinks into the duvet, covering her loneliness.

HOW DO WE RECOGNIZE EMOTIONAL HUNGER? AND WHAT DO WE DO WITH IT?

The identification process consists of seven main stages:

- **Stage A- Identifying the emotional hunger**

Identifying emotional hunger can be elusive, since emotional hunger often disguises itself as physical hunger. We can recognize it by simple technical examination by asking these questions: when did we eat before? Were we full? What did we eat? And so on. Differential diagnosis. Another method is to use the hunger and satiation scale. If our level of hunger is five or higher, the hunger is obviously not physical and we are facing emotional hunger. Emotional hunger is not a bad thing. And we don't have to run away from it or fight it. But the ability to recognize it can give us the choice of how to handle it.

- **Stage B- Identifying the emotion behind the hunger**

In this stage we will focus on identifying the emotion at the root of the hunger. We will often discover that it is difficult to recognize, whether from fear of seeing and knowing it or from a long winded difficulty of repressing and avoiding emotions. There is a full range of emotions and situations which arouse emotional hunger. Any emotion can cause it. Happy or sad ones alike. In this stage we will identify the emotion. Is it frustration, loneliness, fear, or happiness?

- **Stage C- Accepting the emotion**

Making the emotion legitimate may be the most important part in the process of coping with emotional eating. In order to do this we must acknowledge the nature of our emotions and their habit of coming and going. Their ability to affect and manage our behavior. Mindfulness, the ability to be in the here and now with awareness that lacks judgment, criticism, and evaluation, has a principal role in handling emotions. Observing emotions and accepting them provides a refreshing twist from the usual attempts which involve removing, repressin,g and dimming them. Using it helps us see emotions as a small part of the present, of the current experience.

- **Stage D- Identifying judgmental thoughts**

Emotions are often followed by an automatic need to eat. Be it due to the difficulty to feel the emotions or the difficulty of knowing that we are feeling emotional hunger, which is labelled as something illegitimate, that we shouldn't give into or act from. This situation brings judgmental and accusatory thoughts, like "Don't surrender to the binge eating " and encourages us to avoid eating altogether. It is important to recognize these Diet Language thoughts, because this is what can halt the automatic way we react to them.

- **Stage E- The trap between emotion and food**

We find ourselves in a trap, between feeling the emotion and eating it. If we chose to try and run from them by eating them, they may quiet down for a while but they'll still exist. And here we are, "stuck" with both our initial emotions and the critical thoughts and emotions about the unconstrained eating that follows them.

- **Stage F- The ability to let go brings the ability to choose**

We see the emotions on the one hand and the need to avoid feeling them on the other. We are also aware of the possibility of using food as a wonderful method of avoidance, but we also know it's avoidance, which is usually effective only in the short-term. We are thus able to utilize our ability to let it old habits go and choose new ones.

- **Stage G- The choice**

Choosing is an empowering position. There is something logical and free about it, which chooses each time whether to eat emotion or whether to be in it.

  - **Being with the emotion**- This is the ability to give it room to be. To feel it, to experience it. This way eating will stay regular. The emotion will not arouse hunger and won't become a problem to escape or avoid. It will be what it is.
  - **Eating the emotion**- This type of eating is eating out of choice and acknowledging the need to eat the emotion. Even if we have begun eating it when we're not really physically hungry, it is likely that the eating will be done without it becoming a binge. Because it is occurring with inner license, it is no longer eating that is full of guilt and judgment. It will balance in its way later in the day.

If so, once we have allowed emotional eating to exist and let it be, we have turned it into a normal action. We have made the struggle against it redundant. We have validated its existence. Not because it's fun to encounter this type of eating and not because we encourage it, but because it is what it is. By legitimizing it we have taken its power.

> *We can be with our emotions but we can also eat them*

BEING WITH EMOTIONS

Emotions are in tight correlation with our thoughts and behaviors. They can easily become a painful and harmful cycle. Coping with them is a challenge.

MINDFULNESS AND AWARENESS OF EMOTIONS

In order to be with our emotions we must acknowledge their nature. Their habit of coming and going and their ability to affect and run our lives. Keeping a journal is one of the methods of developing emotional mindfulness. In addition to logging the emotion, we should also note the way in which we acted following it and try to document the effectiveness of the response in the short term and in the long term. The emotion log can help us identify all of our emotions, but specifically those which have become chronic. Is the way we behave effective? Is it beneficial? In the short-term? In the long-term? It seems that managing ourselves by these emotions is not always effective, but avoiding feeling them may also be harmful.

Mindfulness, the ability to be in the here and now with awareness that lacks judgment, criticism and, evaluation, has a principal role in handling emotions.

The following exercises will serve us in our journey if we have chosen to be with the emotion rather than eat it. They will allow us to make the emotions present and allow them to come and go, as they do anyway.

- **Exercise- Observing emotions**

The following exercise makes use of mindfulness techniques with the purpose of seeing the emotions and describing them:

- o Focus on your breathing
- o Notice and describe how you feel inside your body
- o Note and describe the emotion
- o Note if the emotion is intensifying or fading away
- o Describe every new emotion or any change in its quality
- o Note any need to block emotion
- o Note the urge to act
- o Note the thoughts of judgment (about yourselves, others, emotion) and let them go
- o Go on observing until the emotion changes or goes away
- o End again with conscious breathing exercises

- **Exercise- Describing emotions**

Try describing an emotion you are feeling right now. It can be a pleasant emotion or an unpleasant one. If you are finding it difficult to identify what you are feeling right now, try to use an emotion you have felt recently. An emotion you can recall easily. Try to be specific in describing it (Sad? Depressed? Sorry? Regretful? Ashamed? Empty? Guilty?).

After you have identified the emotion, write it at the top of a piece of paper. Using your imagination, draw what the emotion looks like. Try to imagine what sound it makes. Then try to describe an action that would be fitting for this emotion.

Try to focus yourselves on identifying the intensity of the emotion and how it is manifested. For instance: "I feel very anxious and I can feel my heart beating.".

Try to describe all of the sensations that you feel in your body following this specific emotion.

Now add the thoughts that accompany the emotion. For instance, "The emotion raises in me a thought that says..." it is important that you distinguish the difference between thought and emotion. For instance, if you feel confident, the thought that accompanies the emotion can be "Today I have the energy to go to an online dating site and try to meet a partner."

- **Exercise- In and out**

Close your eyes and take a deep breath. Try to notice what is happening inside your body. Observe each pleasant experience. At the same time, try to locate any pain or strain, but don't let your mind get stuck on this point.

Do you notice any other sensations like heat, cold, pressure? Note your breathing. Be aware of the sensations in your feet, where they touch the floor. Or in your pelvis, if you're sitting down. After a minute or two of looking inward, open your eyes and turn your attention to what you hear, see, smell. Try to shift from one sensation to another. Look at the colors and shapes around you and allow yourself to notice sounds like a ticking clock, the sound of the refrigerator, or the humming of the air conditioner. After a minute or two close your eyes again and return to looking inward. Try to notice other sensations that you have not noticed before. After a minute, open your eyes and look around you again. At the end of the second round, take a few moments to recall the experience you have just been through. Where were you most comfortable? When do your thoughts run away?

- **Mindfulness of emotions exercise**
  - Watch your emotions and label them. Note how intense they are and to what extent are other emotions mixed up in them.

- o Observe your breathing. Try to pay attention to the diaphragm, to the air coming in and out.
- o When the thoughts appear, label them and let them go. Return to your breathing and your internal state.
- o Let your mind expand while acknowledging all of the space surrounding you. Include your feelings, your breathing, the sensations in your body and the experience and note if this is outside your body or inside it.
- o Let yourselves hold the emotion in its entirety in your breathing, your body and the senses that surround you.
- o Stay with this complex of emotions until the initial emotion eases away like a receding wave.

- **Mindfulness exercise- Revealing emotions**

Take three deep breaths. Note how the breathing feels along your throat, the way the air fills the lungs and how it pushes down on the diaphragm. As you breathe slowly, especially note how you feel in your stomach and chest area. Note your neck, shoulders, and face.

Now notice how you are feeling. Keep your attention focused on the emotion until you feel you've had enough. Describe the emotion to yourself. Name it. Note its intensity. Find the words to describe this intensity. Note if the emotion is intensifying or fading away. If the emotion was a wave, what point of the wave are you on now? Note any change that occurs in them.. Are there other emotions that are starting to rise like waves? Describe each one of them. Keep watching and try to find words that will describe the change in the intensity of emotions and in their quality. While you continue observing, you might notice a need to block the emotion, to push it aside. This is normal, but try to go on observing it. Describe to yourself what you are feeling, and the changes that take place.

Try to see what it means not to act out of your

emotions, not to avoid them, and not to urge them. Only to be aware of their existence without acting out of them. Remind yourself that this is a wave which passes like endless other emotions in life. Waves come and go. Watch the wave and let it pass at its own pace. If judgment appears, about you or others, note this and let it go. Stay attentive of your emotions for a while more.

If they change, let them change. Describe to yourself what you are feeling. Go on observing them until the emotions change or fade away. Finish the exercise with a few deep, mindful breaths. Count your breaths and focus on the experience of each and every breath. And then open your eyes.

- **Mindfulness exercise- Awareness of emotions**

Observe your emotions, watch the air enter through the nose and exit through the mouth. Note how your lungs fill with air and empty out again. After four or five breaths, turn your attention to how you are feeling in this exact moment. Watch the emotion closely. How would you describe it? Try labeling it. Continue to observe the emotion and while you do so go on describing what you see.

Try to see the nuances of it. Does it meet other emotions? If so, what are they? For instance, if you're feeling sadness, is it mixed with a certain anxiety or fear? Note the intensity of the emotion and how it changes as you watch it. Try to discover the way in which the emotion lifts, changes its quality, its intensity.

When you observe your emotion, you will surely recognize the thoughts and physical sensations that accompany it or other interruptions which are attempting to divert you from focusing on it.. This is normal. Try your best to return your gaze to the emotion you are observing. Stay in it until you watch it grow, change, and disappear.

Now see your breathing again, watch the air enter through the nose and exit through the mouth. Note how your lungs fill with air and empty again. Repeat this four-five times. Now slowly open your eyes.

- **Exercise - Nonjudgmental or critical mindfulness of emotions**

Try to focus on your emotions and the air entering your throat. Note the ribs rising and falling and the diaphragm narrowing and expanding. After 4-5 deep breaths, watch the emotion surging inside you. If you cannot recognize, it try to imagine a recent event that has spurred an emotional reaction within you. Try to notice as many details as you can about this event.

Breathe deeply. Note the emotions coursing into your body. Are the emotions located in the chest, the shoulders, the face, the head? Do you feel them in your legs, your arms? Note the physical sensations that are attached to them, and their power. Are they growing stronger or weaker? Are they pleasant or painful? Try to name the emotion and describe it.

Note your thoughts. Are you thinking about the emotions? Do the they trigger judgment about yourself or others?

Try to picture each judgment as:

Leaves floating down the stream

Clouds in the sky

Pop up advertisements that appear on your computer and disappear after two seconds

Choose the image that you relate to the most. Note the judgment and place it on the leaf, the cloud, and so on…and try to let it move on. Keep watching your emotions and when the judgment about them, yourself, or others begins to sprout, try to turn it into something visual and tangible and follow it until it slides out of your line of vision. Remember that the nature of emotions is that they come and go like waves in the ocean. It doesn't matter what you feel, how powerful and painful the emotion is; it will pass. Take a deep, slow breath and accept the emotion as one that lives within you for a certain time and then passes. Note the judgmental thoughts. Watch them and let them go. Let your emotions be as they are and what they are. Let them come and go. This is human and normal. Finish the exercise with a few minutes of deep breaths and then open your eyes.

BEING WITH THEM OR EATING THEM

"If I allowed myself to eat my emotions I'd be 150 kilograms by now," she said. "And if I was able to overcome the need to eat them I would have been thin ages ago. This emotional eating is what stands between me and my thin dream." She was convinced she was right. "Who eats emotions? You can see, feel, experience, run away from them, fear them, but eating them is a different story. Who eats emotions? Only me, beast that I am. Only me, who has no inhibitions," she continued fervently. I smiled and waited quietly. "You know," she said, "I always ate emotions. I like saying that out loud, 'emotion eater'... it has that strange sound of something that's okay, 'eating emotions,' like breathing, like smiling, like loving. Actions that are so routine that we don't even think about them. They are listed in our lexicon of usable, viable, existing words...words... So what do you really mean about me being allowed to eat them without feeling guilty? Without loathing myself for my lack of control?"

"A lot of our suffering stems from our difficulty to accept reality." I replied. "From struggling with it. We find it difficult to understand that not everything has to be like we imagine it should be, and this gap between what the present is and what we'd like it to be hurts us." I raised my eyes, looked at her. "There is no person who doesn't find himself eating without mindfulness of hunger and satiation. Out of feelings, social situations, or just some unclear automatic action. There is also no person who doesn't occasionally get at some chocolate, or cornflakes, or just regular bread and butter. But we think that we have to label every time we eat. Because it seems to us that this is the only way we can gain control over it. Manage it. Police it. But eating is a well-known rebel. It has a hard time confining to the discipline we enforce upon it. It doesn't allow us to control it as much as we want. It is full of cravings and desires and fulfills so many needs. So how did we naively imagine that eating can be so concrete, devoid of emotion, playfulness, desire, and lust?" I paused for breath and went on. "This is what eating is. It is ever-changing, buoyant, surprising, happy, sad, loving, comforting, satiating, empowering, healthy, flattering. Why change this? And can we really?

"And maybe because we have tried to lock it up, it began lashing out? And now we have labeled it with the horrible name of emotional eating. And created a problem."

Ronit, as I have chosen to call her, was paralyzed. "You want to tell me that it's okay? That there's no need to fight this eating that had made me feel so guilty all these years? It's normal to eat when you're sad or happy or just bored?" I nodded and let her mull over my words for a moment.

"The guilty one is the primary suspect," I said. "It is the one who disrupts our minds and our eating and the one berating us in almost every situation. We can choose whether to adhere to it and welcome it or let it go. Because what good does it do us in terms of feeling good, eating healthy, and living? This does not mean 'let's eat' at any time and in any situation, but it does mean that if we have chosen to eat, even of this is not eating out of hunger and satiation, we shouldn't hurt ourselves. Not only because this does us no good, but mostly because it hurts us. Eating, " I explained to her, "was meant to give us more than just nutrition for the body. And we must let it be what it is. We must choose it anew each time."

She breathed a sigh of relief, as if a weight had been lifted off her chest. She sat up, straightened her back and leaned back in the chair, looking more at ease.

"Thank you", she said.

AFTERWORD

"The body is the site on which regimes of discourse inscribe themselves and on which they are undermined,"[69] said Foucault, who was a French philosopher and historian and one of the leading characters in the field of critical theory. It is the greatest battle ground in human history. A struggle between oppressive forces in society and the individual. These are dynamic balances of power in which the body becomes a site in which the discourses inscribe themselves, but at the same time it is also a place which objects to the discourse being built on it. An infinite game is created. A game in which both sides have an interest and the ability to change the situation of the balance of power at any given moment. **The human body is the site of this game.**

In the modern society we live in, the body is disciplined by the tyranny of thinness. Most of the population has adopted disciplinary practices (i.e. different diets) to allegedly help it compel the body to match this ideal. An ideal which has become a disciplinary force, which stands at the head of a global dictatorship which is everywhere and nowhere. A force that does not rely on violence, but its invasion of the body is complete. The individual in our society lives as if he is being tested in any given moment. He internalized the disciplinary glare to such an extent that he becomes his own warden and adopts the restriction of power. Power which in modern society is invasive and has strict social and psychological control. Power that is faceless, concentrated, convincing, and anonymous. Power that has "birthed" a new individuality and within it isolates subjects that discipline themselves. The individual in our society has become a "prisoner" in his own home. He has been robbed of his self and his liberty, and his identity has become defined by his body weight.

The question is, does this body have the strength to create resistance against the sophisticated system of discipline that has enslaved him in diet practices which attempt to police his body? Because the penalties enforced on those who do not succeed in disciplining their body are heavy. Even if most of them are covert, they exist, and seep into all layers of modern day society, maintain the tyranny of the dictatorship and the subordination of the body as if it were an object. Even if the person is not really penalized because he doesn't fit in with the "existing laws of power," he is penalized, day by day, hour by hour, by being constantly at risk of being expelled from society because he "doesn't belong, is worthless, inappropriate" due to his weight. He is always being blamed. The failure to lose weight is awaiting him. And he experiences de-legitimization on a regular basis.

And our body, bowing down to an oppressive eating regime, finds it difficult to free itself. The rebellion against restriction, hunger, pain and self- hatred fails every time. Whether it be in the form of a new diet which promises to make the dream a reality, or in the form of an aggressive intimidation campaign which links health to weight. And whether it be in the form of weight discrimination, which invades all fields of life at work, at home, and in the media.

The fact that a regime is strict does not ensure it will be overthrown, since most people accept these difficulties as necessary and obligatory. Furthermore, there is also no promise that this rebellion will bring liberty, even if there are cells of resistance, taking different forms, like the fat acceptance movements, anti-dieting movements and movements that work towards acceptance of legitimate social differences.

A danger lurks behind attempts at revolution: anti-diet and body acceptance movement are constantly changing and fleeting, and they create rifts in society that run through the individuals themselves, and recut and reshapes them. Is such an evolution indeed freeing, or does it just enforce a different kind of regime that is just as oppressive, supervising and penalizing? In parting from the Diet Language will we truly free ourselves or will we unwittingly start to believe another?

This book was written to be a beacon in the fog blinding the eyes of those who worship the tyranny of thinness. Those who experience the nightmare of failing diets and live an entire life feeling as if they are worth nothing. This book was meant to dispel truths that have long become axioms, dictating social discourse. In many ways this book dares to deny these alleged truths in order to bring us from slavery to freedom. Freedom in which we will allow ourselves to eat with pleasure without having to justify it, where body weight does not run our lives and we are not constantly busy counting calories. This is a type of freedom in which the individual does not subordinate himself to external rules, but dares to be the master of his own body and takes pride in it, so only he can know why he is hungry, how hungry he is and what he most wants to eat. In many ways this book is here to free us from the fear, prohibition and guilt that have stuck to us and return sanity to eating.

I have not tried to present a different method of weight loss or create another kind of regime; I have only tried to look at the existing reality with a critical eye. An eye which can give new perspective and present options for the observer to choose from, whether to adhere to the Diet Language which is the familiar default choice or adhere to this subjective mindfulness, which is the most personal and the most adapted to every different individual.

Any parting, even if we have chosen it, has its sad moments. Moments of missing what was and will never be. That moment before innocence was shattered, that maintained the dream as an ideal that we can and should achieve. A moment after which nothing will be the same again. Dieting will suddenly seem pale and maybe even silly, the mind will empty of thoughts and words of a language that will suddenly sound old fashioned, and the door will close behind it, never to be opened again. Because we will never be able to diet, even if we want to. And new phrases, including mindfulness, hunger, satiation, pleasure, choice and acceptance will enter our lives, and with acceptance on one side and loss on the other, hope will emerge. In it is a life of after and a life of towards. Life promoting health for people of all shapes and sizes, being careful of judging a person because of his weight, respecting others and believing that happiness has no weight.

ABOUT THE AUTHOR

Ayelet Kalter (M.Sc.RD) is the founder and managing director of the "Eating Dialog Center, for treating obesity and eating behaviors". The Center is a pioneer of HEAS principles in Israel. Kalter is also the CEO of the Israeli nonprofit organization for preventing size discrimination.

She is a clinical dietitian with a degree in biochemistry and nutrition from the Hebrew University of Jerusalem, in collaboration with the School of Social Work at Tel-Aviv University.

Kalter studied psychotherapy in the Program of Psycho-dynamic Approaches to Adult Development Comprehension at Tel-Aviv University. She also studied family therapy, group directing and studies at the Israeli Center of Body and Soul Health.

Kalter attends and lectures at conferences both in Israel and abroad. She writes newspaper articles, takes part in radio and television shows and serves as a consultant in her field for firms and institutions. Furthermore, Kalter lectures to M.Sc. nutritionist students at the Faculty of Agriculture, Rehovoth. In the past, she was the chairwoman and spokeswoman of "Atid" - the Association of Clinical Dietitians in Israel.

Ayelet Kalter published 2 books: How Much Does Happiness weigh – on food, body and spirit", Published by Yediot Acharonot Publishing (2005). "All of us are real people – Diet: the most successful failure in the modern era", Published by Rimonim publishing and distributed by Keter (2011).

REMARKS

1. Treating obesity seriously: when recommendations for lifestyle change confront biological adaptations. Lancet Diabetes Endocrinol 2015 Published Online February 12, 2015 http://dx.doi.org/10.1016/S2213-8587(15)00009-1

2. Lelwica, M. M. (2013). The Religion of Thinness: Satisfying the Spiritual Hungers Behind Women's Obsession with Food and Weight. Gurze Books.

3. Mills, S. (2005). Michel Foucault. Resling Publishing (Hebrew). Tel Aviv. 109.

4. Szymborska, W. (2004). Pochwala Snow. Keshev, (Hebrew). 30.

5. Garner, D. M., & Wooley, S. C. (1991). Confronting the failure of behavioral and dietary treatments for obesity. Clinical Psychology Review, 11(6), 729-780.

6. Rosenbaum, M., Leibel, R. L., & Hirsch, J. (1997). Obesity. The New England Journal of Medicine, 337(6), 396-407.

7. Mann, T., Tomiyama, A. J., Westling, E., Lew, A. M., Samuels, B., & Chatman, J. (2007). Medicare's search for effective obesity treatments: diets are not the answer. American Psychologist, 62(3), 220-233.

8. Hughes, V. (2013). The big fat truth. Nature, 497(7450), 428-430.

9. Flegal, K. M., Kit, B. K., Orpana, H., & Graubard, B. I. (2013). Association of all-cause mortality with overweight and obesity using standard body mass index categories: a systematic review and meta-analysis. Jama, 309(1), 71-82.

10. Flegal, K. M., Graubard, B. I., Williamson, D. F., & Gail, M. H. (2005). Excess deaths associated with underweight, overweight, and obesity. Jama, 293(15), 1861-1867.

11. Dorner, T. E., & Rieder, A. (2012). Obesity paradox in elderly patients with cardiovascular diseases. International Journal of Cardiology, 155(1), 56-65.

12. Gruberg, L., Weissman, N. J., Waksman, R., Fuchs, S., Deible, R., Pinnow, E. E, ... & Lindsay, J. (2002). The impact of obesity on the short-term and long-term outcomes after percutaneous coronary intervention: the obesity paradox? Journal of the American College of Cardiology, 39(4), 578-584.

13. Kenchaiah, S., Evans, J. C., Levy, D., Wilson, P. W., Benjamin, E. J., Larson, M. G., ... & Vasan, R. S. (2002). Obesity and the risk of heart failure. New England Journal of Medicine, 347(5), 305-313.

14. Oreopoulos, A., Padwal, R., Kalantar-Zadeh, K., Fonarow, G. C., Norris, C. M., & McAlister, F. A. (2008). Body mass index and mortality in heart failure: a meta-analysis. American Heart Journal, 156(1), 13-22.

15. Uretsky, S., Messerli, F. H., Bangalore, S., Champion, A., Cooper-DeHoff, R. M., Zhou, Q., & Pepine, C. J. (2007). Obesity paradox in patients with hypertension and coronary artery disease. The American Journal of Medicine,120(10), 863-870.

16. Benderly, M., Boyko, V., & Goldbourt, U. (2010). Relation of body mass index to mortality among men with coronary heart disease. The American Journal of Cardiology, 106(3), 297-304.

17. Gaesser, G. A. (2002). Big fat lies. Gurze Books.

18. Ibid.

19. Blake, A., Miller, W.C. & Brown, D.A. (2000). Adiposity does not hinder the fitness response to
   exercise training in obese women. Journal of Sports med phys fitness, 40, 170-177.

20. Wessel, T. R., Arant, C. B., Olson, M. B., Johnson, B. D., Reis, S. E., Sharaf, B. L., ... & Merz, C. N. B. (2004). Relationship of physical fitness vs body mass index with coronary artery disease and cardiovascular events in women. Jama, 292(10), 1179-1187.

21. McAuley, P. A., Sui, X., Church, T. S., Hardin, J. W., Myers, J. N., & Blair, S. N. (2009). The joint effects of cardiorespiratory fitness and adiposity on mortality risk in men with hypertension. American Journal of Hypertension, 22(10), 1062-1069.

22. McAuley, P. A., & Blair, S. N. (2011). Obesity paradoxes. Journal of Sports Sciences, 29(8), 773-782.

23. Szymborska, W. (2004). Pochwala Snow. Keshev, (Hebrew). 137.

24. Parker-Pope, T. A. R. A. (2011). The fat trap. The New York Times.

25. Sumithran, P., Prendergast, L. A., Delbridge, E., Purcell, K., Shulkes, A., Kriketos, A., & Proietto, J. (2011). Long-term persistence of hormonal adaptations to weight loss. New England Journal of Medicine, 365(17), 1597-1604.

26. Rosenbaum, M., Hirsch, J., Gallagher, D. A., & Leibel, R. L. (2008). Long-term persistence of adaptive thermogenesis in subjects who have maintained a reduced body weight. The American Journal of Clinical Nutrition, 88(4), 906-912.

27. Parker-Pope, T. A. R. A. (2011). The fat trap. The New York Times.

28. Neumark-Sztainer, D., Wall, M., Guo, J., Story, M., Haines, J., & Eisenberg, M. (2006). Obesity, disordered eating, and eating disorders in a longitudinal study of adolescents: how do dieters fare 5 years later? Journal of the American Dietetic Association, 106(4), 559-568.

29. Bouchard, C., Tremblay, A., Després, J. P., Nadeau, A., Lupien, P. J., Thériault, G. ... & Fournier, G. (1990). The response to long-term overfeeding in identical twins. New England Journal of Medicine, 322(21), 1477-1482.

30. Parker-Pope, T. A. R. A. (2011). The fat trap. The New York Times.

31. Speliotes, E. K., Willer, C. J., Berndt, S. I., Monda, K. L., Thorleifsson, G., Jackson, A. U., ... & Hoesel, V. (2010). Association analyses of 249,796 individuals reveal

18 new loci associated with body mass index. Nature genetics, 42(11), 937-948.

32. Freathy, R. M., Timpson, N. J., Lawlor, D. A., Pouta, A., Ben-Shlomo, Y., Ruokonen, A., ... & Frayling, T. M. (2008). Common variation in the FTO gene alters diabetes-related metabolic traits to the extent expected given its effect on BMI. Diabetes, 57(5), 1419-1426.

33. Parker-Pope, T. A. R. A. (2011). The fat trap. The New York Times.

34. Timpson, N. J., Emmett, P. M., Frayling, T. M., Rogers, I., Hattersley, A. T., McCarthy, M. I., & Smith, G. D. (2008). The fat mass–and obesity-associated locus and dietary intake in children. The American Journal of Clinical Nutrition, 88(4), 971-978.

35. Peng, S., Zhu, Y., Xu, F., Ren, X., Li, X., & Lai, M. (2011). FTO gene polymorphisms and obesity risk: a meta-analysis. BMC Medicine, 9(1), 71.

36. Keys, A., Brožek, J., Henschel, A., Mickelsen, O., & Taylor, H. L. (1950). The biology of human starvation. (2 vols).

37. Parker-Pope, T. A. R. A. (2011). The fat trap. The New York Times.

38. Ibid.

39. Orwell, G. (1996). 1984. Am Oved, (Hebrew), Tel Aviv. *200.*

40. Puhl, R. M., & Heuer, C. A. (2010). Obesity stigma: important considerations for public health. Health, 24, 252.

41. Musher-Eizenman, D. R., Holub, S. C., Miller, A. B., Goldstein, S. E., & Edwards-Leeper, L. (2004). Body size stigmatization in preschool children: The role of control attributions. Journal of Pediatric Psychology, 29(8), 613-620.

42. Puhl, R. M., Luedicke, J., & Heuer, C. (2011). Weight- based victimization toward overweight adolescents: Observations and reactions of peers. Journal of School Health, 81(11), 696-703.

43. Puhl, R. M., Luedicke, J., & DePierre, J. A. (2013). Parental concerns about weight-based victimization in youth. Childhood Obesity, 9(6), 540-548.

44. Eisenberg, M. E., Neumark-Sztainer, D., & Story, M. (2003). Associations of weight-based teasing and emotional well-being among adolescents. Archives of Pediatrics & Adolescent Medicine, 157(8), 733-738.

45. Heuer, C. A., McClure, K. J., & Puhl, R. M. (2011). Obesity stigma in online news: a visual content analysis. Journal of Health Communication, 16(9), 976-987.

46. Puhl, R. M., & Brownell, K. D. (2006). Confronting and coping with weight stigma: an investigation of overweight and obese adults. Obesity, 14(10), 1802-1815.

47. Smith, C. A., Schmoll, K., Konik, J., & Oberlander, S. (2007). Carrying Weight for the World: Influence of Weight Descriptors on Judgments of Large- Sized

Women. Journal of Applied Social Psychology, 37(5), 989-1006.

48. Sheets, V., & Ajmere, K. (2005). Are romantic partners a source of college students' weight concern?. Eating Behaviors, 6(1), 1-9.

49. Puhl, R. M., & Brownell, K. D. (2006). Confronting and coping with weight stigma: an investigation of overweight and obese adults. Obesity, 14(10), 1802-1815.

50. Foster, G. D., Wadden, T. A., Makris, A. P., Davidson, D., Sanderson, R. S., Allison, D. B., & Kessler, A. (2003). Primary care physicians' attitudes about obesity and its treatment. Obesity Research, 11(10), 1168-1177.

51. Puhl, R., Wharton, C., & Heuer, C. (2009). Weight bias among dietetics students: implications for treatment practices. Journal of the American Dietetic Association, 109(3), 438-444.

52. Swift, J. A., Hanlon, S., El Redy, L., Puhl, R. M., & Glazebrook, C. (2013). Weight bias among UK trainee dietitians, doctors, nurses and nutritionists. Journal of Human Nutrition and Dietetics, 26(4), 395-402.

53. Sutin, A. R., & Terracciano, A. (2013). Perceived weight discrimination and obesity. PLoS One, 8(7), e70048.

54. Pessoa, F.A.N. (2004). Da Mais Alta Janela. Carmel, (Hebrew) Jerusalem. 145.

55. Harrison, J. (2013). Know Reality, Find Peace. Simply Meditate. 21.

56. Antonovsky, A. (1996). The salutogenic model as a theory to guide health promotion. Health Promotion International, 11(1), 11-18.

57. Hoffmann, Y. (2007). Radical Zen. Babel, (Hebrew), Tel Aviv. 1.

58. Pessoa, F.A.N. (2004). Da Mais Alta Janela. Carmel, (Hebrew) Jerusalem. 124.

59. Ibid. 125.

60. Pessoa, F. (2002). The Book of Disquiet, edited and translated by Richard Zenith. Penguin.

61. Pessoa, F.A.N. (2004). Da Mais Alta Janela. Carmel, (Hebrew) Jerusalem. 142.

62. Yovel, Y. (2011). Acceptance and Commitment, in Marom, S. Gilboa-Schechtman, E. Mor, N. Meijers, J. ed. Cognitive Behavioral Therapy for Adults. Dyonon of Provok House. (Hebrew). 374.

63. Mishol, A. (2000). Dream Notebook. Even Hoshen to Arts, (Hebrew). 7.

64. Pelled, E. (2007). Raising Goodness All Around, Buddhism, Meditation, Psychotherapy. Resling, (Hebrew).

65. Chabris, C. Simons, D. (2012). The Invisible Gorilla. Kineret, Zmora-Bitan, Dvir, (Hebrew).

66. Raveh, D. (2010). Philosophical Threads in Patanjali's Yoga. Hakibbutz Hameuchad, (Hebrew), Tel Aviv. 104.

67. McKay, M., Fanning, P., & Ona, P. Z. (2011). Mind and emotions: A universal treatment for emotional disorders. New Harbinger Publications

68. McKay, M., Fanning, P., & Ona, P. Z. (2011). Mind and emotions: A universal treatment for emotional disorders. New Harbinger Publications

69. Mills, S. (2005). Michel Foucault. Resling Publishing (Hebrew). Tel Aviv. 109.

CHOSEN BIBLIOGRAPHY

Obesity paradox

Aronson, D., Nassar, M., Goldberg, T., Kapeliovich, M., Hammerman, H., & Azzam, Z. S. (2010). The impact of body mass index on clinical outcomes after acute myocardial infarction. International Journal of Cardiology, 145(3), 476-480.

Barclay, L. (2010). Waist to height ratio may predict cardiometabolic risk in normal weight children CME. BMC Pediatr, 10, 73.

Benderly, M., Boyko, V., & Goldbourt, U. (2010). Relation of body mass index to mortality among men with coronary heart disease. The American Journal of Cardiology, 106(3), 297-304.

Benderly, M., Boyko, V., & Goldbourt, U. (2010). Relation of body mass index to mortality among men with coronary heart disease. The American Journal of Cardiology, 106(3), 297-304.

Blake, A., Miller, W. C., & Brown, D. A. (2000). Adiposity does not hinder the fitness response to exercise training in obese women. The Journal of Sports Medicine and Physical Fitness, 40(2), 170-177.

Curtis, J. P., Selter, J. G., Wang, Y., Rathore, S. S., Jovin, I. S., Jadbabaie, F., ... & Krumholz, H. M. (2005). The obesity paradox: body mass index and outcomes in patients with heart failure. Archives of internal medicine, 165(1), 55-61.

Dorner, T. E., & Rieder, A. (2012). Obesity paradox in elderly patients with cardiovascular diseases. International Journal of Cardiology, 155(1), 56-65.

Dorner, T. E., & Rieder, A. (2012). Obesity paradox in elderly patients with cardiovascular diseases. International journal of cardiology, 155(1), 56-65.

Ferreira, I., & Stehouwer, C. D. (2012). Obesity paradox or inappropriate study designs? Time for life-course epidemiology. Journal of hypertension, 30(12), 2271-2275.

Flegal, K. M., Graubard, B. I., Williamson, D. F., & Gail, M. H. (2005). Excess deaths associated with underweight, overweight, and obesity. Jama, 293(15), 1861-1867.

Flegal, K. M., Graubard, B. I., Williamson, D. F., & Gail, M. H. (2007). Cause-specific excess deaths associated with underweight, overweight, and obesity.Jama, 298(17), 2028-2037.

Flegal, K. M., Kit, B. K., Orpana, H., & Graubard, B. I. (2013). Association of all-cause mortality with overweight and obesity using standard body mass index categories: a systematic review and meta-analysis. Jama, 309(1), 71-82.

Flicker, L., McCaul, K. A., Hankey, G. J., Jamrozik, K., Brown, W. J., Byles, J. E., & Almeida, O. P. (2010). Body mass index and survival in men and women aged 70 to 75. Journal of the American Geriatrics Society, 58(2), 234-241.

Franzosi, M. G. (2006). Should we continue to use BMI as a cardiovascular risk factor? The Lancet, 368(9536), 624-625.

Gaesser, G. (2002). Big Fat Lies. Carlsbad.

Gronniger, J. T. (2006). A semiparametric analysis of the relationship of body mass index to mortality. American Journal of Public Health, 96(1), 173.

Gruberg, L., Weissman, N. J., Waksman, R., Fuchs, S., Deible, R., Pinnow, E. E., ... & Lindsay, J. (2002). The impact of obesity on the short-term and long-term outcomes after percutaneous coronary intervention: the obesity paradox?.Journal of the American College of Cardiology, 39(4), 578-584.

Habbu, A., Lakkis, N. M., & Dokainish, H. (2006). The obesity paradox: fact or fiction? The American journal of cardiology, 98(7), 944-948.

Hu, G., Jousilahti, P., Antikainen, R., Katzmarzyk, P. T., & Tuomilehto, J. (2010). Joint effects of physical activity, body mass index, waist circumference, and waist-to-hip ratio on the risk of heart failure. Circulation, 121(2), 237-244.

Hughes, V. (2013). The big fat truth. Nature, 497(7450), 428-430.

Johnson, N. P., Wu, E., Bonow, R. O., & Holly, T. A. (2008). Relation of exercise capacity and body mass index to mortality in patients with intermediate to high risk of coronary artery disease. The American Journal of Cardiology,102(8), 1028-1033.

Karelis, A. D., Faraj, M., Bastard, J. P., St-Pierre, D. H., Brochu, M., Prud'homme, D., & Rabasa-Lhoret, R. (2005). The metabolically healthy but obese individual presents a favorable inflammation profile. The Journal of Clinical Endocrinology & Metabolism, 90(7), 4145-4150.

Kenchaiah, S., Evans, J. C., Levy, D., Wilson, P. W., Benjamin, E. J., Larson, M. G., ... & Vasan, R. S. (2002). Obesity and the risk of heart failure. New England Journal of Medicine, 347(5), 305-313.

Kenchaiah, S., Pocock, S. J., Wang, D., Finn, P. V., Zornoff, L. A., Skali, H., ... & Solomon, S. D. (2007). Body mass index and prognosis in patients with chronic heart failure insights from the candesartan in heart failure: Assessment of reduction in mortality and morbidity (CHARM) Program. Circulation, 116(6), 627-636.

Lavie, C. J. (2014). The Obesity Paradox: when thinner means sicker and heavier means healthier. Penguin.

Lavie, C. J., Milani, R. V., & Ventura, H. O. (2009). Obesity and Cardiovascular DiseaseRisk Factor, Paradox, and Impact of Weight Loss. Journal of the American College of Cardiology, 53(21), 1925-1932.

Matheson, E. M., King, D. E., & Everett, C. J. (2012). Healthy lifestyle habits and mortality in overweight and obese individuals. The Journal of the American Board of Family Medicine, 25(1), 9-15.

McAuley, P. A., & Blair, S. N. (2011). Obesity paradoxes. Journal of Sports Sciences, 29(8), 773-782.

McAuley, P. A., Smith, N. S., Emerson, B. T., & Myers, J. N. (2012). The obesity paradox and cardiorespiratory fitness. Journal of obesity, 2012.

Oreopoulos, A., Padwal, R., Kalantar-Zadeh, K., Fonarow, G. C., Norris, C. M., & McAlister, F. A. (2008). Body mass index and mortality in heart failure: a meta-analysis. American Heart Journal, 156(1), 13-22.

Orpana, H. M., Berthelot, J. M., Kaplan, M. S., Feeny, D. H., McFarland, B., & Ross, N. A. (2010). BMI and mortality: results from a national longitudinal study of Canadian adults. Obesity, 18(1), 214-218..

Rexrode, K. M., Carey, V. J., Hennekens, C. H., Walters, E. E., Colditz, G. A., Stampfer, M. J., ... & Manson, J. E. (1998). Abdominal adiposity and coronary heart disease in women. Jama, 280(21), 1843-1848.

Romero-Corral, A., Montori, V. M., Somers, V. K., Korinek, J., Thomas, R. J., Allison, T. G., ... & Lopez-Jimenez, F. (2006). Association of bodyweight with total mortality and with cardiovascular events in coronary artery disease: a systematic review of cohort studies. The Lancet, 368(9536), 666-678.

Schmidt, M. D., Dwyer, T., Magnussen, C. G., & Venn, A. J. (2010). Predictive associations between alternative measures of childhood adiposity and adult cardio-metabolic health. International Journal of Obesity, 35(1), 38-45.

Speliotes, E. K., Willer, C. J., Berndt, S. I., Monda, K. L., Thorleifsson, G., Jackson, A. U., ... & Hoesel, V. (2010). Association analyses of 249,796 individuals reveal 18 new loci associated with body mass index. Nature Genetics, 42(11), 937-948.

Uretsky, S., Messerli, F. H., Bangalore, S., Champion, A., Cooper-DeHoff, R. M., Zhou, Q., & Pepine, C. J. (2007). Obesity paradox in patients with hypertension and coronary artery disease. The American journal of medicine, 120(10), 863-870.

Wessel, T. R., Arant, C. B., Olson, M. B., Johnson, B. D., Reis, S. E., Sharaf, B. L., ... & Merz, C. N. B. (2004). Relationship of physical fitness vs body mass index with coronary artery disease and cardiovascular events in women. Jama, 292(10), 1179-1187.

Widlansky, M. E., Sesso, H. D., Rexrode, K. M., Manson, J. E., & Gaziano, J. M. (2004). Body mass index and total and cardiovascular mortality in men with a history of cardiovascular disease. Archives of internal medicine, 164(21), 2326-2332.

Zajacova, A., Dowd, J. B., & Burgard, S. A. (2011). Overweight adults may have the lowest mortality—do they have the best health? American journal of epidemiology, kwq382.

Childhood obesity

Denny, K. N., Loth, K., Eisenberg, M. E., & Neumark-Sztainer, D. (2013). Intuitive eating in young adults. Who is doing it, and how is it related to disorder eating behaviors? Appetite, 60, 13-19.

Field, A. E., Austin, S. B., Taylor, C. B., Malspeis, S., Rosner, B., Rockett, H. R., ... & Colditz, G. A. (2003). Relation between dieting and weight change among preadolescents and adolescents. Pediatrics, 112(4), 900-906.

Kopelman, P. G., Caterson, I. D., & Dietz, W. H. (Eds.). (2009). Clinical obesity in adults and children. John Wiley & Sons.

Ogden, C. L., Carroll, M. D., Curtin, L. R., Lamb, M. M., & Flegal, K. M. (2010). Prevalence of high body mass index in US children and adolescents, 2007-2008. Jama, 303(3), 242-249.

Ogden, C. L., Carroll, M. D., Kit, B. K., & Flegal, K. M. (2012). Prevalence of obesity and trends in body mass index among US children and adolescents, 1999-2010. Jama, 307(5), 483-490.

Tanofsky-Kraff, M., Cohen, M. L., Yanovski, S. Z., Cox, C., Theim, K. R., Keil, M., ... & Yanovski, J. A. (2006). A prospective study of psychological predictors of body fat gain among children at high risk for adult obesity. Pediatrics, 117(4), 1203-1209.

Mindful Eating

Adams, C. E., McVay, M. A., Kinsaul, J., Benitez, L., Vinci, C., Stewart, D. W., & Copeland, A. L. (2012). Unique relationships between facets of mindfulness and eating pathology among female smokers. Eating behaviors, 13(4), 390-393.

Albers, S. (2009). Eat, drink, and be mindful: how to end your struggle with mindless eating and start savoring food with intention and joy. New Harbinger Publications.

Albers, S. (2010). Using Mindful Eating to treat food restriction: A case study. Eating disorders, 19(1), 97-107.

Albers, S. (2012). Eating mindfully: How to end mindless eating and enjoy a balanced relationship with food. New Harbinger Publications.

Alberts, H. J., Mulkens, S., Smeets, M., & Thewissen, R. (2010). Coping with food cravings. Investigating the potential of a mindfulness-based intervention. Appetite, 55(1), 160-163.

Augustus-Horvath, C. L., & Tylka, T. L. (2011). The acceptance model of intuitive eating: a comparison of women in emerging adulthood, early adulthood, and middle adulthood. Journal of Counseling Psychology, 58(1), 110.

Baer, R. A., Fischer, S., & Huss, D. B. (2005). Mindfulness-based cognitive therapy applied to binge eating: A case study. Cognitive and Behavioral Practice, 12(3), 351-358.

Bahl, S., Milne, G. R., Ross, S. M., & Chan, K. (2013). Mindfulness: A Long-Term Solution for Mindless Eating by College Students. Journal of Public Policy & Marketing, 32(2), 173-184.

Bays, J. C. (2009). Mindful Eating. Shambhala Publications.

Beshara, M., Hutchinson, A. D., & Wilson, C. (2013). Does mindfulness matter? Everyday mindfulness, Mindful Eating and self-reported serving size of energy dense foods among a sample of South Australian adults. Appetite, 67, 25-29.

Bush, H. E., Rossy, L., Mintz, L. B., & Schopp, L. (2013). Eat for Life: A Work Site Feasibility Study of a Novel Mindfulness-Based Intuitive Eating Intervention. American Journal of Health Promotion, 28(6), 380-388.

Chabris, C. F., & Simons, D. J. (2011). The invisible gorilla: And other ways our intuitions deceive us. Random House LLC.

Cowdrey, F. A., & Park, R. J. (2012). The role of experiential avoidance, rumination and mindfulness in eating disorders. Eating behaviors, 13(2), 100-105.

Dalen, J., Smith, B. W., Shelley, B. M., Sloan, A. L., Leahigh, L., & Begay, D. (2010). Pilot study: Mindful Eating and Living (MEAL): weight, eating behavior, and psychological outcomes associated with a mindfulness-based intervention for people with obesity. Complementary therapies in medicine, 18(6), 260-264.

Forman, E. M., Butryn, M. L., Hoffman, K. L., & Herbert, J. D. (2009). An open trial of an acceptance-based behavioral intervention for weight loss. Cognitive and Behavioral Practice, 16(2), 223-235.

Forman, E. M., Hoffman, K. L., McGrath, K. B., Herbert, J. D., Brandsma, L. L., & Lowe, M. R. (2007). A comparison of acceptance-and control-based strategies for coping with food cravings: An analog study. Behaviour research and therapy, 45(10), 2372-2386.

Framson, C., Kristal, A. R., Schenk, J. M., Littman, A. J., Zeliadt, S., & Benitez, D. (2009). Development and validation of the Mindful Eating Questionnaire.Journal of the American Dietetic Association, 109(8), 1439-1444.

Gravel, K., Deslauriers, A., Watiez, M., Dumont, M., Dufour Bouchard, A. A., & Provencher, V. (2014). Sensory-based nutrition pilot intervention for women. Journal of the Academy of Nutrition and Dietetics, 114(1), 99-106.

Gravel, K., Ouellet St-Hilaire, G., Deslauriers, A., Watiez, M., Dumont, M., Dufour Bouchard, A. A., & Provencher, V. (2014). Effect of sensory-based intervention on the increased use of food-related descriptive terms among restrained eaters. Food Quality and Preference, 32, 271-276.

Hawks, S., Merrill, R. M., & Madanat, H. N. (2004). The intuitive eating scale: Development and preliminary validation. American Journal of Health Education,35(2), 90-99.

Hong, P. Y., Lishner, D. A., & Han, K. H. (2014). Mindfulness and eating: An experiment examining the effect of mindful raisin eating on the enjoyment of sampled food. Mindfulness, 5(1), 80-87.

Jacobs, J., Cardaciotto, L., Block-Lerner, J., & McMahon, C. (2012). A pilot study of a single-session training to promote Mindful Eating. Advances in Mind-Body Medicine, 27(2), 18-23.

Kabatznick, R. (1998). The zen of eating: Ancient answers to modern weight problems. Penguin.

Kristeller, J., Wolever, R. Q., & Sheets, V. (2014). Mindfulness-based eating awareness training (MB-EAT) for binge eating: A randomized clinical trial.Mindfulness, 5(3), 282-297.

Kristeller, J., Wolever, R. Q., & Sheets, V. (2014). Mindfulness-based eating awareness training (MB-EAT) for binge eating: A randomized clinical trial. Mindfulness, 5(3), 282-297.

Kristeller, J.L. (2014). Eat, drink, be mindful. Mindful, 2 (1), 66.

Kristeller, J.L. and Epel, E. (2014). Mindful Eating and mindless eating. In A. le, C.T. Ngnoumen, & E.J. Langer (Eds.). The Wiley Blackwell Handbook of Mindfulness. Vol.2, Ch. 47, pp. 913-931

Lillis, J., Hayes, S. C., Bunting, K., & Masuda, A. (2009). Teaching acceptance and mindfulness to improve the lives of the obese: a preliminary test of a theoretical model. Annals of Behavioral Medicine, 37(1), 58-69.

Madden, C. E., Leong, S. L., Gray, A., & Horwath, C. C. (2012). Eating in response to hunger and satiety signals is related to BMI in a nationwide sample of 1601 mid-age New Zealand women. Public health nutrition, 15(12), 2272-2279.

McKay, M., Fanning, P., & Ona, P. Z. (2011). Mind and emotions: A universal treatment for emotional disorders. New Harbinger Publications.

Miller, C. K., Kristeller, J. L., Headings, A., Nagaraja, H., & Miser, W. F. (2012). Comparative effectiveness of a Mindful Eating intervention to a diabetes self-management intervention among adults with type 2 diabetes: a pilot study. Journal of the Academy of Nutrition and Dietetics, 112(11), 1835-1842.

Miller, C. K., Kristeller, J. L., Headings, A., Nagaraja, H., & Miser, W. F. (2012). Comparative effectiveness of a Mindful Eating intervention to a diabetes self-management intervention among adults with type 2 diabetes: a pilot study. Journal of the Academy of Nutrition and Dietetics, 112(11), 1835-1842.

Moon, A., & Berenbaum, H. (2009). Emotional awareness and emotional eating. Cognition and Emotion, 23(3), 417-429.

Moor, K. R., Scott, A. J., & McIntosh, W. D. (2013). Mindful Eating and its relationship to body mass index and physical activity among university students. Mindfulness, 4(3), 269-274.

Schaefer, J. T., & Magnuson, A. B. (2014). A Review of Interventions that Promote Eating by Internal Cues. Journal of the Academy of Nutrition and Dietetics, 114(5), 734-760.

Schoenefeld, S. J., & Webb, J. B. (2013). Self-compassion and intuitive eating in college women: Examining the contributions of distress tolerance and body image acceptance and action. Eating Behaviors, 14(4), 493-496.

Smith, T., & Hawks, S. R. (2006). Intuitive eating, diet composition, and the meaning of food in healthy weight promotion. American Journal of Health Education, 37(3), 130-136.

Taitz, J. (2012). End Emotional Eating: Using Dialectical Behavior Therapy Skills to Cope with Difficult Emotions and Develop a Healthy Rela. New Harbinger Publications.

Teixeira, P. J., Patrick, H., & Mata, J. (2011). Why we eat what we eat: the role of autonomous motivation in eating behavior regulation. Nutrition Bulletin, 36(1), 102-107.

Timmerman, G. M., & Brown, A. (2012). The Effect of a Mindful Restaurant Eating Intervention on Weight Management in Women. Journal of Nutrition Education and Behavior, 44(1), 22-28.

Tylka, T. L., & Kroon Van Diest, A. M. (2013). The Intuitive Eating Scale–2: Item refinement and psychometric evaluation with college women and men. Journal of Counseling Psychology, 60(1), 137-153.

Urbszat, D., Herman, C. P., & Polivy, J. (2002). Eat, drink, and be merry, for tomorrow we diet: effects of anticipated deprivation on food intake in restrained and unrestrained eaters. Journal of Abnormal Psychology, 111(2), 396-401.

Wansink, B., Just, D. R., & Payne, C. R. (2009). Mindless eating and healthy heuristics for the irrational. The American Economic Review, 165-169.

Fat Discrimination

Almeida, L., Savoy, S., & Boxer, P. (2011). The role of weight stigmatization in cumulative risk for binge eating. Journal of Clinical Psychology, 67(3), 278-292.

Andreyeva, T., Puhl, R. M., & Brownell, K. D. (2008). Changes in perceived weight discrimination among Americans, 1995–1996 through 2004–2006. Obesity, 16(5), 1129-1134.

Brownell, K. D. (Ed.). (2005). Weight bias: Nature, consequences, and remedies. Guilford Press.

Danielsdottir, S., O'Brien, K. S., & Ciao, A. (2010). Anti-fat prejudice reduction: a review of published studies. Obesity facts, 3(1), 47-58.

Farrell, A. E. (2011). Fat shame: Stigma and the fat body in American Culture. NYU Press.

Foster, G. D., Wadden, T. A., Makris, A. P., Davidson, D., Sanderson, R. S., Allison, D. B., & Kessler, A. (2003). Primary care physicians' attitudes about obesity and its treatment. Obesity Research, 11(10), 1168-1177.

Hatzenbuehler, M. L., Keyes, K. M., & Hasin, D. S. (2009). Associations between perceived weight discrimination and the prevalence of psychiatric disorders in the general population. Obesity, 17(11), 2033-2039.

Heuer, C. A., McClure, K. J., & Puhl, R. M. (2011). Obesity stigma in online news: a visual content analysis. Journal of Health Communication, 16(9), 976-987.

Muennig, P. (2008). The body politic: the relationship between stigma and obesity-associated disease. BMC Public Health, 8(1), 128.

Musher-Eizenman, D. R., Holub, S. C., Miller, A. B., Goldstein, S. E., & Edwards-Leeper, L. (2004). Body size stigmatization in preschool children: The role of control attributions. Journal of Pediatric Psychology, 29(8), 613-620.

O'Hara, L., & Gregg, J. (2012). Human rights casualties from the "war on obesity": Why focusing on body weight is inconsistent with a human rights approach to health. Fat Studies, 1(1), 32-46.

O'Reilly, C., & Sixsmith, J. (2012). From Theory to Policy: Reducing Harms Associated with the Weight-Centered Health Paradigm. Fat Studies, 1(1), 97-113.

Pearl, R. L., Puhl, R. M., & Brownell, K. D. (2012). Positive media portrayals of obese persons: Impact on attitudes and image preferences. Health Psychology, 31(6), 821.

Puhl, R. M., & Brownell, K. D. (2006). Confronting and coping with weight stigma: an investigation of overweight and obese adults. Obesity, 14(10), 1802-1815.

Puhl, R. M., & Heuer, C. A. (2009). The stigma of obesity: a review and update. Obesity, 17(5), 941-964.

Puhl, R. M., & Heuer, C. A. (2009). The stigma of obesity: a review and update. Obesity, 17(5), 941-964.

Puhl, R. M., & Heuer, C. A. (2010). Obesity stigma: important considerations for public health. Health, 24, 252.

Puhl, R. M., Andreyeva, T., & Brownell, K. D. (2008). Perceptions of weight discrimination: prevalence and comparison to race and gender discrimination in America. International Journal of Obesity, 32(6), 992-1000.

Puhl, R. M., Andreyeva, T., & Brownell, K. D. (2008). Perceptions of weight discrimination: prevalence and comparison to race and gender discrimination in America. International Journal of Obesity, 32(6), 992-1000.

Puhl, R., & Brownell, K. D. (2001). Bias, discrimination, and besity. Obesity Research, 9(12), 788-805.

Puhl, R., Peterson, J. L., & Luedicke, J. (2012). Fighting obesity or obese persons? Public perceptions of obesity-related health messages.International Journal of Obesity, 37(6), 774-782 .

Puhl, R., Wharton, C., & Heuer, C. (2009). Weight bias among dietetics students: implications for treatment practices. Journal of the American Dietetic Association, 109(3), 438-444.

Saguy, A. C., & Ward, A. (2011). Coming Out as Fat Rethinking Stigma. Social Psychology Quarterly, 74(1), 53-75.

Schwartz, M. B., Chambliss, H. O. N., Brownell, K. D., Blair, S. N., & Billington, C. (2003). Weight bias among health professionals specializing in obesity. Obesity research, 11(9), 1033-1039.

Sheets, V., & Ajmere, K. (2005). Are romantic partners a source of college students' weight concern? Eating Behaviors, 6(1), 1-9.

Sikorski, C., Luppa, M., Kaiser, M., Glaesmer, H., Schomerus, G., König, H. H., & Riedel-Heller, S. G. (2011). The stigma of obesity in the general public and its implications for public health-a systematic review. BMC public health, 11(1), 661.

Smith, C. A., Schmoll, K., Konik, J., & Oberlander, S. (2007). Carrying Weight for the World: Influence of Weight Descriptors on Judgments of Large-Sized Women. Journal of Applied Social Psychology, 37(5), 989-1006.

Stone, O., & Werner, P. (2012). Israeli dietitians' professional stigma attached to obese patients. Qualitative Health Research, 22(6), 768-776.

Stone, O., & Werner, P. (2012). Israeli dietitians' professional stigma attached to obese patients. Qualitative Health Research, 22(6), 768-776.

Sutin, A. R., & Terracciano, A. (2013). Perceived weight discrimination and obesity. PLoS One, 8(7), e70048.

Sutin, A. R., & Terracciano, A. (2013). Perceived weight discrimination and obesity. PLoS One, 8(7), e70048.

Swift, J. A., Hanlon, S., El-Redy, L., Puhl, R. M., & Glazebrook, C. (2013). Weight bias among UK trainee dietitians, doctors, nurses and nutritionists. Journal of Human Nutrition and Dietetics, 26(4), 395-402.

Tirosh, Y. (2013). The Right to Be Fat. Yale Journal of Health Policy, Law, and Ethics, 12(2), 2.

Tsenkova, V. K., Carr, D., Schoeller, D. A., & Ryff, C. D. (2011). Perceived weight discrimination amplifies the link between central adiposity and nondiabetic glycemic control (HbA1c). Annals of Behavioral Medicine, 41(2), 243-251.

Wang, S. S., Brownell, K. D., & Wadden, T. A. (2004). The influence of the stigma of obesity on overweight individuals. International journal of obesity, 28(10), 1333-1337.

Mindfulness and Acceptance

Baer, R.A. (2005). Mindfulness-based treatment approaches: Clinician's Guide to Evidence Base and Applications. Academic Press.

Biderman, S. (1980). Early Buddhism. Ministry of Defense Israel.

Biserman, S. (1995). Indian philosophy. Ministry of Defense Israel.

Daubenmier, J., Kristeller, J., Hecht, F. M., Maninger, N., Kuwata, M., Jhaveri, K., ... & Epel, E. (2011). Mindfulness intervention for stress eating to reduce cortisol and abdominal fat among overweight and obese women: an exploratory randomized controlled study. Journal of Obesity, 2011.

Eifert, G. H., & Forsyth, J. P. (2005). Acceptance and commitment therapy for anxiety disorders. Oakland, CA: New Harbinger.

Eifert, G. H., & Forsyth, J. P. (2005). Acceptance and commitment therapy for anxiety disorders. Oakland, CA: New Harbinger.

Gethin, R. (1998). The foundations of Buddhism. Oxford University Press.

Harris, R. (2007). The happiness trap: Stop struggling, start living. Exisle Publishing.

Harris, R. (2009). ACT with love. Oakland, CA: New Harbinger.

Harris, R. (2009). ACT made simple: An easy-to-read primer on acceptance and commitment therapy. New Harbinger Publications.

Hayes, S. C., & Wilson, K. G. (1993). Some applied implications of a contemporary behavior-analytic account of verbal events. Behavior Analyst, 16, 283-301.

Hayes, S. C., & Strosahl, K. D. (Eds.). (2004). A practical guide to acceptance and commitment therapy. Springer.

Hayes, S. C., Follette, V. M., & Linehan, M. (Eds.). (2004). Mindfulness and acceptance: Expanding the cognitive-behavioral tradition. Guilford Press.

Hayes, S. C., & Smith, S. (2005). Get out of your mind and into your life: The new acceptance and commitment therapy. New Harbinger Publications.
Hayes, S. C., Luoma, J. B., Bond, F. W., Masuda, A., & Lillis, J. (2006). Acceptance and commitment therapy: Model, processes and outcomes. Behaviour Research and Therapy, 44(1), 1-25.

Hayes, S. C., Strosahl, K. D., & Wilson, K. G. (1999). Acceptance and commitment therapy: An experiential approach to behavior change. Guilford Press.

Hayes, S. C., Strosahl, K. D., & Wilson, K. G. (2011). Acceptance and commitment therapy: The process and practice of mindful change. Guilford Press.

Hayes, S. C., Strosahl, K. D., & Wilson, K. G. (2011). Acceptance and commitment therapy: The process and practice of mindful change. Guilford Press.

Kabat-Zinn, J. (1994). Wherever you go, there you are: Mindfulness meditation in everyday life. Hyperion.

Kabat-Zinn, J. (1996). Mindfulness meditation: What it is, what it isn't, and its role in health care and medicine. Comparative and psychological study on meditation. Netherlands: Eburon.

Kabat-Zinn, J. (2003). Mindfulness-based interventions in context: past, present, and future. Clinical psychology: Science and practice, 10(2), 144-156.

Kornfield, J. (2009). The wise heart: A guide to the universal teachings of Buddhist psychology. Random House LLC.

Labbé, E. E. (2011). Psychology moment by moment: A guide to enhancing your clinical practice with mindfulness and meditation. New Harbinger Publications.

Lillis, J., & Hayes, S. C. (2008). Measuring avoidance and inflexibility in weight related problems. International Journal of Behavioral Consultation and Therapy, 4(1), 30-40.

Lillis, J., Hayes, S. C., Bunting, K., & Masuda, A. (2009). Teaching acceptance and mindfulness to improve the lives of the obese: a preliminary test of a theoretical model. Annals of Behavioral Medicine, 37(1), 58-69.

Luoma, J. B., Hayes, S. C., & Walser, R. D. (2007). Learning ACT: An Acceptance & Commitment Therapy skills-training manual for therapists. New Harbinger Publications.

McKay, M., Wood, J. C., & Brantley, J. (2007). The dialectical behavior therapy skills workbook. Oakland: New Harbinger.

Orsillo, S. M., & Roemer, L. (2011). The mindful way through anxiety: Break free from chronic worry and reclaim your life. Guilford Press.

Pearson, A. N., Heffner, M., & Follette, V. M. (2010). Acceptance & Commitment Therapy for Body Image Dissatisfaction: A Practitioner's Guide to Using Mindfulness, Acceptance & Values-based Behavior Change Strategies. New Harbinger Publications.

Peled, E. (2007). Raising goodness all around – Buddhism. Meditation. Psychotherapy. Resling.

Raveh, D. (2010). Philosophical threads in Patanjaliws Yoga. Hakibbutz Hameuchad.

Roemer, L., & Orsillo, S. M. (2009). Mindfulness- and acceptance-based behavioral therapies in practice. New York: Guilford Press.

Ruiz, F. J. (2010). A review of Acceptance and Commitment Therapy (ACT) empirical evidence: Correlational, experimental psychopathology, component and outcome studies. International Journal of Psychology and Psychological Therapy, 10(1), 125-162.

Ruiz, F. J. (2010). A review of Acceptance and Commitment Therapy (ACT) empirical evidence: Correlational, experimental psychopathology, component and outcome studies. International Journal of Psychology and Psychological Therapy, 10(1), 125-162.

Siegel, D. J. (2010). The mindful therapist. A Clinician's Guide to Mindsight and chotherapy.

Siegel, R. D. (2009). The mindfulness solution: Everyday practices for everyday problems. Guilford Press.

Strosahl, K., Wilson, K. G., Bissett, R. T., Polusny, M. A., Dykstra, T. A., Batten, S. V., & Mccurry, S. M. (2004). Measuring experiential avoidance: A preliminary test of a working model. The Psychological Record, 54, 553-578.

Yovel, Y. (2011). Acceptance and commitment, in Marom, S., Gilboa-Schechterman, E., Mor, N., Meijers, J., ed. Cognitive behavioral therapy for adults – Therapeutic principles. Dyonon.

Weight Focus Approaches – Obesity and the Diets Failure

Birch, L. L., Fisher, J. O., & Davison, K. K. (2003). Learning to overeat: maternal use of restrictive feeding practices promotes girls' eating in the absence of hunger. The American Journal of Clinical Nutrition, 78(2), 215-220.

Bosomworth, N. J. (2012). The downside of weight loss Realistic intervention in body-weight trajectory. Canadian Family Physician, 58(5), 517-523.

Cecil, J. E., Tavendale, R., Watt, P., Hetherington, M. M., & Palmer, C. N. (2008). An obesity-associated FTO gene variant and increased energy intake in children. New England Journal of Medicine, 359(24), 2558-2566.

Field, A. E., Austin, S. B., Taylor, C. B., Malspeis, S., Rosner, B., Rockett, H. R., ... & Colditz, G. A. (2003). Relation between dieting and weight change among preadolescents and adolescents. Pediatrics, 112(4), 900-906.

Freathy, R. M., Timpson, N. J., Lawlor, D. A., Pouta, A., Ben-Shlomo, Y., Ruokonen, A., ... & Frayling, T. M. (2008). Common variation in the FTO gene alters diabetes-related metabolic traits to the extent expected given its effect on BMI. Diabetes, 57(5), 1419-1426.

Gregg, E. W., Gerzoff, R. B., Thompson, T. J., & Williamson, D. F. (2004). Trying to lose weight, losing weight, and 9-year mortality in overweight US adults with diabetes. Diabetes Care, 27(3), 657-662.

Hill, A. J. (2004). Does dieting make you fat? British Journal of Nutrition, 92(S1), S15-S18.

Jansen, E., Mulkens, S., & Jansen, A. (2007). Do not eat the red food! Prohibition of snacks leads to their relatively higher consumption in children. Appetite, 49(3), 572-577.

Keys, A., Brožek, J., Henschel, A., Mickelsen, O., & Taylor, H. L. (1950). The biology of human starvation. (2 vols).

Kruger, J., Galuska, D. A., Serdula, M. K., & Jones, D. A. (2004). Attempting to lose weight: specific practices among US adults. American Journal of Preventive Medicine, 26(5), 402-406.

Mann, T., Tomiyama, A. J., Westling, E., Lew, A. M., Samuels, B., & Chatman, J. (2007). Medicare's search for effective obesity treatments: diets are not the answer. American Psychologist, 62(3), 220.

Neumark-Sztainer, D., Wall, M., Guo, J., Story, M., Haines, J., & Eisenberg, M. (2006). Obesity, disordered eating, and eating disorders in a longitudinal study of adolescents: how do dieters fare 5 years later?. Journal of the American Dietetic Association, 106(4), 559-568.

Neumark-Sztainer, D., Wall, M., Haines, J., Story, M., & Eisenberg, M. E. (2007). Why does dieting predict weight gain in adolescents? Findings from project EAT-II: a 5-year longitudinal study. Journal of the American Dietetic Association, 107(3), 448-455.

Owen, L. (2012). Living fat in a thin-centric world: Effects of spatial discrimination on fat bodies and selves. Feminism & Psychology, 22(3) 290–306.

Parker-Pope, T. A. R. A. (2011). The fat trap. The New York Times.

Peng, S., Zhu, Y., Xu, F., Ren, X., Li, X., & Lai, M. (2011). FTO gene polymorphisms and obesity risk: a meta-analysis. BMC Medicine, 9(1), 71.

Polivy, J., Coleman, J., & Herman, C. P. (2005). The effect of deprivation on food cravings and eating behavior in restrained and unrestrained eaters. International Journal of Eating Disorders, 38(4), 301-309.

Rosenbaum, M., Hirsch, J., Gallagher, D. A., & Leibel, R. L. (2008). Long-term persistence of adaptive thermogenesis in subjects who have maintained a reduced body weight. The American journal of clinical nutrition, 88(4), 906-912.

Scott, M. L., Nowlis, S. M., Mandel, N., & Morales, A. C. (2008). The effects of reduced food size and package size on the consumption behavior of restrained and unrestrained eaters. Journal of Consumer Research, 35(3), 391-405.

Shils, M. E., & Shike, M. (Eds.). (2006). Modern nutrition in health and disease. Lippincott Williams & Wilkins.

Sumithran, P., Prendergast, L. A., Delbridge, E., Purcell, K., Shulkes, A., Kriketos, A., & Proietto, J. (2011). Long-term persistence of hormonal adaptations to weight loss. New England Journal of Medicine, 365(17), 1597-1604.

Wade, T., George, W. M., & Atkinson, M. (2009). A randomized controlled trial of brief interventions for body dissatisfaction. Journal of Consulting and Clinical Psychology, 77(5), 845.

Health Focus Approaches

Antonovsky, A. (1996). The salutogenic model as a theory to guide health promotion. Health Promotion International, 11(1), 11-18.

Appel, L. J., Moore, T. J., Obarzanek, E., Vollmer, W. M., Svetkey, L. P., Sacks, F. M., ... & Harsha, D. W. (1997). A clinical trial of the effects of dietary patterns on blood pressure. New England Journal of Medicine, 336(16), 1117-1124.

Bacon, L., & Aphramor, L. (2011). Weight science: evaluating the evidence for a paradigm shift. Nutrition Journal, 10(9), 2-13.

Bacon, L., Keim, N. L., Van Loan, M. D., Derricote, M., Gale, B., Kazaks, A., & Stern, J. S. (2002). Evaluating a" non-diet' wellness intervention for improvement of metabolic fitness, psychological well-being and eating and activity behaviors. International Journal of Obesity, 26, 854-865.

Bacon, L., Stern, J. S., Van Loan, M. D., & Keim, N. L. (2005). Size acceptance and intuitive eating improve health for obese, female chronic dieters. Journal of the American Dietetic Association, 105(6), 929-936.

Bradshaw, A. J., Horwath, C. C., Katzer, L., & Gray, A. (2010). Non-dieting group interventions for overweight and obese women: what predicts non-completion and does completion improve outcomes? Public Health Nutrition, 13(10), 1622-1628.

Brown, L. B. (2009). Teaching the "health at every size" paradigm benefits future fitness and health professionals. Journal of Nutrition Education and Behavior, 41(2), 144-145.

Campos, P., Saguy, A., Ernsberger, P., Oliver, E., & Gaesser, G. (2006). The epidemiology of overweight and obesity: public health crisis or moral panic? International Journal of Epidemiology, 35(1), 55-60.

Carrier, K. M., Steinhardt, M. A., & Bowman, S. (1994). Rethinking traditional weight management programs: a 3-year follow-up evaluation of a new approach. The Journal of Psychology, 128(5), 517-535.

Carroll, S., Borkoles, E., & Polman, R. (2007). Short-term effects of a non-dieting lifestyle intervention program on weight management, fitness, metabolic risk, and psychological well-being in obese premenopausal females with the metabolic syndrome. Applied Physiology, Nutrition, and Metabolism, 32(1), 125-142.

Ciliska, D. (1998). Evaluation of two nondieting interventions for obese women. Western Journal of Nursing Research, 20(1), 119-135.

Clifford, D., Ozier, A., Bundros, J., Moore, J., Kreiser, A., Neyman Morris, M. (2015). Impact of non-diet approaches on attitudes, behaviors, and health outcomes: a systematic review. Journal of Nutrition Education and Behavior, 47(2), 143-155.

Dulloo, A. G., Montani, J. P. (2015). Pathways from dieting to weight regain, to obesity and to the metabolic syndrome: an overview. Obesity Reviews, 16(S1), 1-6.

Dulloo, A. G., Jacquet, J., Montani, J. P., & Schutz, Y. (2015). How dieting makes the lean fatter: from a perspective of body composition autoregulation through adipostats and proteinstats awaiting discovery. Obesity Reviews, 16(S1), 25-35.

Gagnon-Girouard, M. P., Bégin, C., Provencher, V., Tremblay, A., Mongeau, L., Boivin, S., & Lemieux, S. (2010). Psychological impact of a "Health-at-Every-Size" intervention on weight-preoccupied overweight/obese women. Journal of Obesity, 1-12.

Goodrick, G. K., Poston II, W. S. C., Kimball, K. T., Reeves, R. S., & Foreyt, J. P. (1998). Nondieting versus dieting treatment for overweight binge-eating women. Journal of Consulting and Clinical Psychology, 66(2), 363.

Gregg, J. A., O'Hara, L., & Barnes, M. (2014). Health promotion: a critical salutogenic science. International Journal of Social Work and Human Services Practice, 2(6), 283-290.

Kalter, A. (2005). How much does happiness weigh? Miskal.

Kalter, A. (2011). We are all real people. Rimonim.

Kulick, D., & Meneley, A. (2005). Fat: The anthropology of an obsession. Penguin.

Lelwica, M. M. (2013). The Religion of Thinness: Satisfying the Spiritual Hungers Behind Women's Obsession with Food and Weight. Gurze Books.

Matz, J., & Frankel, E. (2014). Beyond a Shadow of a Diet: The Therapist's Guide to Treating Compulsive Eating Disorders. Second ed, Routledge.

Miller, W. C., & Jacob, A. V. (2001). The health at any size paradigm for obesity treatment: the scientific evidence. Obesity Reviews, 2(1), 37-45.

Montani, J. P., Schutz, Y., & Dulloo, A. G. (2015). Dieting and weight cycling as risk factors for cardiometabolic diseases: who is really at risk? Obesity Reviews, 16(S1), 7-18.

Neumark-Sztainer, D., Paxton, S. J., Hannan, P. J., Haines, J., & Story, M. (2006). Does body satisfaction matter? Five-year longitudinal associations between body satisfaction and health behaviors in adolescent females and males. Journal of Adolescent Health, 39(2), 244-251.

Niemeier, H. M., Craighead, L. W., Pung, M. A., & Elder, K. A. (2002, November). Reliability, validity and sensitivity to change of the Preoccupation with Eating Weight, and Shape Scale. In Annual meeting of the Association of the Advancement of Behavior Therapy, Reno, NV.

Orbach, S. (1998). Fat is a Feminist Issue: The Anti-diet Guide for Women+ Fat is a Feminist (No. 2). Random House.

Provencher, V., Bégin, C., Tremblay, A., Mongeau, L., Boivin, S., & Lemieux, S. (2007). Short-Term Effects of a "Health-At-Every-Size" Approach on Eating Behaviors and Appetite Ratings. Obesity, 15(4), 957-966.

Provencher, V., Bégin, C., Tremblay, A., Mongeau, L., Boivin, S., & Lemieux, S. (2007). Short-Term Effects of a "Health-At-Every-Size" Approach on Eating Behaviors and Appetite Ratings. Obesity, 15(4), 957-966.

Provencher, V., Bégin, C., Tremblay, A., Mongeau, L., Corneau, L., Dodin, S., ... & Lemieux, S. (2009). Health-at-every-size and eating behaviors: 1-year follow-up results of a size acceptance intervention. Journal of the American Dietetic Association, 109(11), 1854-1861.

Robison, J., Putnam, K., & McKibbin, L. (2007). Health At Every Size: a compassionate, effective approach for helping individuals with weight-related concerns--Part II. AAOHN Journal: official journal of the American Association of Occupational Health Nurses, 55(5), 185-192.

Stearns, P. N. (2002). Fat history: Bodies and beauty in the modern west. NYU Press.

Tylka, T. L., Annunziato, R. A., Burgard, D., Daníelsdóttir, S., Shuman, E., Davis, C., & Calogero, R. M. (2014). The Weight-inclusive versus weight-normative approach to health: evaluating the evidence for prioritizing well-being over weight loss. Journal of Obesity, July, 1-18.

Wolf, N. (1991). The beauty myth: How images of beauty are used against women. Random House.

www.ingramcontent.com/pod-product-compliance
Lightning Source LLC
Chambersburg PA
CBHW030426290526
45786CB00001B/150

* 9 7 8 1 5 1 1 6 1 1 2 1 3 *